The Hidden Secrets *of* EFT

The Hidden Secrets of EFT

CAROL PRENTICE

Published through Elevation Publishing

Copyright © 2011 by Carol Prentice. All rights reserved.

Published by Elevation Publishing

FIRST EDITION 2011

No part of this publication may be reproduced, stored, shared or transmitted in any form (physical or electronic) without prior written permission from the author.

1st ed.

ISBN-13:   978-1461171232
ISBN-10:   1461171237

Disclaimer:

By reading this book you assume full responsibility for how you choose to use this content. The information contained in this book is provided for educational purposes only and is not intended to replace qualified medical advice.

For further information please contact:

Email: support@TheHiddenSecretsofEFT.com

Web: www.TheHiddenSecretsofEFT.com

Layout and typesetting by Mara Dower (maradower@gmail.com)

Cover design by Panisa Soison (p.s.cnx@hotmail.com)

Author Photo courtesy of © Brock University

I have chosen to dedicate this book to my mother, Wanda, who has lived with mental illness for many years. She has inspired me to help others heal and guide them to cultivate a sound mind with a positive outlook on life—more than she could possibly ever know.

~ Carol Prentice

www.TheHiddenSecretsofEFT.com

Contents

How to Read this Book	1, 3
Part 1: EFT Introduction	5
Part II: Basic EFT Technique	17
Part III: Advanced EFT Techniques	29
Part IV: The Hidden Secrets of EFT	53
Skyrocket Your Self-esteem	55
Free Yourself From Fear and Anxiety For Good	75
Ridding the Toxic Relationships in Your Life and Connecting to Love	97
Release Your Emotions, Release Your Fat	123
Busting the Top 8 Smoking Myths—So You Can Stop Smoking Permanently	145
How to Upgrade Your Thoughts to Increase Your Bank Balance	173
Creating Your New Identity	235
Final Thoughts	269

The Author

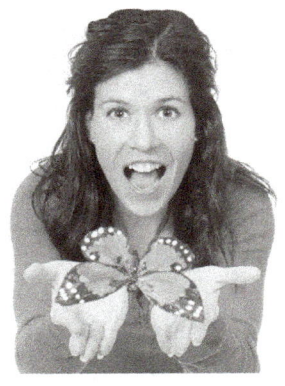

Carol Prentice

With over 10 years of experience, Carol Prentice is known for her exquisite blend of Western Psychology and Eastern healing traditions as she guides each of her clients closer to experiencing profound peace in their lives.

With university degrees in Psychology and Social Work, she has cultivated a deep understanding of how we create our reality from the inside out.

As a certified Emotional Freedom Technique Therapist and a Yoga Instructor, Carol has also developed a comprehension of the body's energy system and a unique approach to healing the mind and body.

Carol approaches every Emotional Freedom Technique private session, workshop and retreat with compassion, brilliance and the intention to heal from the heart.

www.TheHiddenSecretsofEFT.com

www.TheHiddenSecretsofEFT.com

How To Read This Book

How to Read This Book

To give you a solid grounding of how to use Emotional Freedom Technique (EFT), I recommend you familiarize yourself with Part I and Part II as a minimum. You can then dive into Part IV and use EFT to address whatever area you would like relief from.

If you get stuck, you can refer to Part III for advanced techniques and trouble-shooting. Or you can read Part III before Part IV so you already have this knowledge, should you need it.

There is no time limit in which you must learn this new technique. Starting with one session a day, is probably a reasonable pace for most people.

www.TheHiddenSecretsofEFT.com

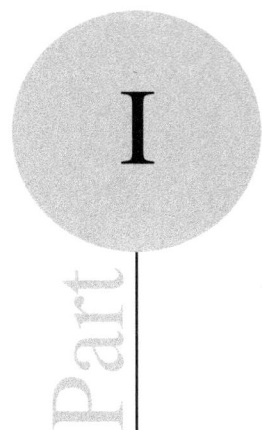

EFT Introduction

EFT Introduction

EFT or *Emotional Freedom Technique*, is a popular therapy that can treat a wide range of emotional, mental and physical issues.

It is based on the Meridian System as used by the Chinese for thousands of years. EFT is popularly described as "psychological acupuncture, but without the needles".

This book will take you through the background, techniques and applications of EFT.

Do you have any long-standing emotions that are negatively affecting your life and would like to clear once and for all? Do you harbor resentment, anger or consistent negativity?

Do you suffer from any form of physical pain on a frequent basis? Do you experience regular headaches, a stiff neck or regular bouts of flu?

Are you mentally healthy, or do you feel depressed, anxious or constantly fearful?

You may have tried everything you can think of to free yourself of the emotional, physical or mental pain. But in every direction you turn, you may have come up against something that prevents you from breaking free.

If you feel at the end of your tether and are tired of being a slave to your emotional, physical or mental pain—you have come to the right book.

www.TheHiddenSecretsofEFT.com

I don't know of any drug that can help heal the real root problem. Drugs only act as a band-aid and in many cases can make the original problem worse.

There is another way. I invite you to step off the downward ladder of despair and try a new way of healing.

It is my belief that any pain we experience has an emotional connection, and that when your emotional balance is restored, your physical and mental health will naturally heal too.

EFT is an easy, fast and effective way to heal your emotional health. Let's take a look now at the origins of EFT...

EFT History

EFT is one of the many forms of Meridian Energy Therapies; the history of which can be traced back throughout the world, thousands of years ago.

EFT originated from Thought Field Therapy (TFT), which was discovered by psychologist Dr. Roger Callahan in the 1980's. Callahan had been studying acupuncture and kinesiology and both their influences can still be seen.

While Callahan developed the basic concept and structure of EFT, it was Stamford engineer, Gary Craig who had the vision to refine it and make it accessible to everyone.

Gary Craig developed EFT in the early 1990's and he, along with many other therapists working in this field, began to realize the broader possibilities for EFT.

EFT still continues to be refined to this day.

As a therapeutic technique there is nothing else to equal EFT's simplicity and effectiveness. Many experienced therapists report typical success rates of 80% to 95% for many conditions.

Whilst the immediate history of EFT is short, its future looks to be much longer.

How Does EFT Work?

To be honest, nobody knows for certain how EFT produces the results it does; however, there are a few theories…

EFT uses the end points of the 12 major meridian channels and the 2 governing vessels found in Chinese Medicine.

There's the belief that thoughts and/or memories can trigger a disruption in the body's energy system. This disruption is experienced as emotional, physical or mental pain within the body.

It appears that whilst focusing on a specific problem, and tapping on the meridian points, any disruptions and emotional pain being worked on are cleared. EFT restores and rebalances the body, returning it to normal.

The Apex Effect

On occasion, after practising EFT to heal a particular problem, you may think you never had the problem in the first place. Or if you did, that it simply went away of its own accord and had nothing to do with EFT.

It could be further heightened by a general disbelief that EFT could ever work in the first place.

This is known as the Apex Effect.

For this reason, it's important you write down whatever problem you're treating, and also the intensity level (how strongly you feel the pain surrounding this problem) before starting your EFT treatment.

Luckily, you don't have to believe EFT will work for it to produce results for you.

Keeping a Record

Keeping a diary is a great way to record your EFT sessions you conduct and to physically observe your progress.

Before using EFT, write down exactly how you feel and how your current problem is affecting you. How do you feel? What triggers your feelings?

Once you've finished your EFT session, write down how you immediately feel, wait two or three days, and note down again how you feel.

Document the changes you are noticing. Do you feel happier when you think about your old problem? Does it feel so long ago that it no longer feels a part of you? Write down anything you feel.

As you continue to use EFT, you'll see a direct correlation in the improvement of your health. This will be a positive pattern that will increase your confidence in using EFT.

After a year or so, you will be able to look back over your progress and see the evidence of EFT working its magic. You may not remember all the problems you used to have or how badly they affected your life (because of the Apex Effect), but your diary will.

Psychological Reversal

A concept developed by Dr. Roger Callahan as part of *Thought Field Therapy* (TFT), Psychological Reversal is thought to happen when the energy flow in the body becomes reversed (although there are many acupuncturists that refute that's even possible).

I believe something different.

To me, Psychological Reversal is more like an energetic muscle spasm—one that's created originally to help protect the mental, emotional or energetic bodies—but now no longer serves a beneficial purpose.

However you choose to interpret the nature of psychological reversal, the effect is the same.

When psychological reversal is present, it means there is a subconscious part of you that doesn't want to overcome a problem. This is despite you consciously (or even desperately) wanting to overcome the problem.

The part of us that still needs and wants to hold onto an issue will resist and sabotage any changes you attempt, making it impossible to overcome your problem.

Your subconscious mind will always win—until you dissolve the seemingly illogical and ridiculous reasons that explain why you are holding onto your problem.

As a therapist previously practising other techniques, I remember seeing clients who should have responded to treatment, but didn't. There was no logical reason for this, except for psychological reversal. It gives an explanation as to why their healing was blocked.

Without using muscle testing it is hard to know whether someone is reversed or not and to what degree. Thankfully, EFT takes care of this problem by treating everyone as if they are reversed.

(The fact that EFT treats psychological reversal regardless, is probably one of the main contributing factors to its huge success rate.)

It is even harder for us to let go of our problem if secondary gain is present. (Secondary gain is when you benefit indirectly from having your problem.)

Protecting secondary gains is one of the most common reasons why you might be psychologically reversed.

I once had a client who was chronically ill. After some initial tapping we discovered that a part of her didn't want to get well because she loved the undivided attention and care she received from her husband.

Another client came to see me unable to shift excess weight after trying unsuccessfully for five years. We found out a part of her didn't want to lose weight as she didn't want to be rejected by her family and close friends who were also overweight.

I could fill a whole book with examples where secondary gain has played a big part in their psychological reversal, but I'm sure you've grasped the concept.

If you're honest about how your problem benefits you, there is often a whole host of hidden benefits you will uncover.

Perhaps you need your problem because you feel safe, comfortable and familiar with it? Who would you be without your problem? How does it define you? Is your problem part of your identity?

What are you trying to prove by having this problem? Is there someone you blame for having this problem? Can you forgive them?

If your problem no longer existed what would this mean for you? Would you lose something or somebody? Is your problem a convenient cover up that is preventing you from dealing with something else in your life?

Do you need this problem to serve as an excuse for why your life is messed up?

Would your life be dull without the existence of your problem? Would you feel lonely, unloved and invisible without the drama in your life?

All your subconscious mind is trying to do is protect you — because it recognizes there are many benefits to keeping the problem. It protects you from losing these benefits the easiest way it knows how—by making it impossible for you to let go of the problem.

The good news is, you can identify and uncover the underlying benefits to your problem—and safely let go of your problem for good.

It's an empowering feeling to understand why you haven't been able to heal from your problem; and to know that you don't have to hang onto your problem in order to receive those benefits anymore.

When You Need a Therapist

Like any therapy, you'll find a small minority of people who get little or no benefit from EFT. If you are one of these people, it's important you don't blame EFT—there may be a whole gamut of reasons for it not benefiting you.

For most of you, this book is more than you will need in learning how to practice EFT.

But if you cannot make any progress by yourself, this is where you will benefit from an experienced EFT Therapist. Do not be afraid to seek qualified assistance if you get stuck.

Sometimes, just having someone else tap for you and guide you through the process is enough to make a difference.

Or sometimes your emotions may be too overwhelming to deal with (such as severe trauma or abuse) and in these cases an EFT Therapist would be best to help you with "soft approach techniques".

They know of extra tapping points and advanced techniques to help you with more tricky situations. EFT Therapists are trained to understand what may be missing and where you may be going wrong.

www.TheHiddenSecretsofEFT.com

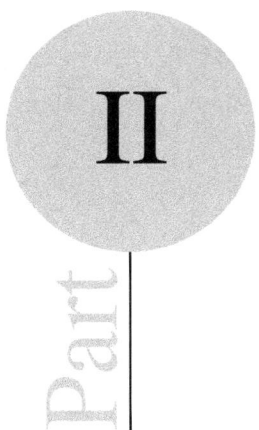

Basic EFT Technique

Setup Phrase

The first thing we do in EFT is identify your problem and create a setup phrase. The basic formula for this is:

"Even though I have this (PROBLEM), I deeply and completely love and accept myself."

So for example if you had a headache you would say:

"Even though I have this headache, I deeply and completely love and accept myself"

The key to an effective setup phrase is to be *as specific as possible*. While you can work on more general issues, it will take you much longer. Focusing on an exact time, event or emotion, and naming anyone involved, attains much quicker and more profound results.

With time you will learn to develop setup phrases that target the problem very quickly. When working on physical pain, try to name its location and describe its feeling. For example, *"this throbbing pain just behind my left eye."*

Reminder Phrase

This is a simple phrase used to help remain focused on your problem and prevent your mind from wandering. So in the example of a headache, the reminder phrase would simply be *"this headache"*.

With more involved pain that may have a long description, you can either repeat the whole phrase, or abbreviate it. For example, *"this sharp shooting pain up the left side of my leg whenever I try to bend over,"* can simply be shortened to *"sharp shooting pain".*

The important point is to remain focused on where you would feel the pain.

Measuring the Effect

To make sure the process of EFT is working, it is important to monitor your progress.

Before you start, close your eyes and tune into your problem. For strong emotions that feel overwhelming, go slowly and tap a lot before focusing on your problem.

Measure the intensity of your problem on a scale of 0–10. This value is known as the Subjective Units of Distress (SUD) level, or otherwise known as your intensity level, where 0 is no anxiety or intensity and 10 is extreme distress, panic, anxiety and highest intensity.

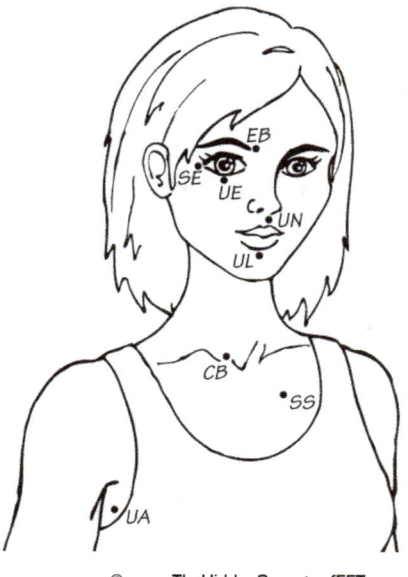

© www.TheHiddenSecretsofEFT.com

In EFT, we look to reduce this level to a 0. This may not always be possible as sometimes there are underlying problems that still need to be worked on.

Face and Body Points

Following, are the locations of the face and body tapping points used in EFT therapy in order of tapping:

1. **SS**: Sore Spot—a tender spot 2-3 inches down and across from the top of the sternum.
2. **EB**: EyeBrow—located at the beginning of the eyebrow on the bone of the eye socket.
3. **SE**: Side of Eye—on the bone at the edge of the eye.
4. **UE**: Under Eye—just under the eye on the bone centered with the pupil.
5. **UN**: Under Nose—found on the crease between the nose and upper lip.
6. **UL**: Under Lip—between the lower lip and chin.
7. **CB**: Collar Bone—where the collarbone meets the sternum.
8. **UA**: Under Arm—located at the side of the body, in line with the nipple on a man or where the bra strap runs on a woman.

www.TheHiddenSecretsofEFT.com

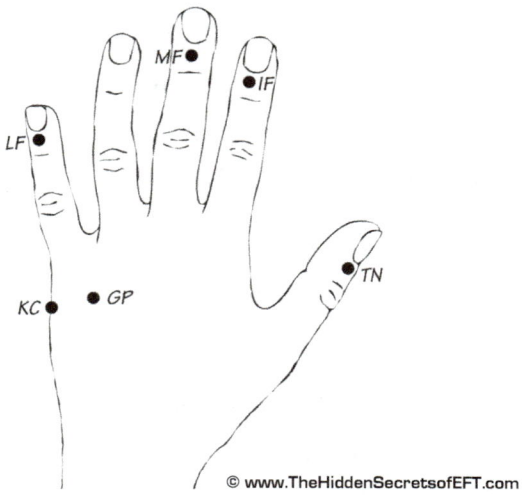

Hand Points

Following, are the tapping points for the hand:

9. **TN**: Thumb Nail—tapping the edge point at the base of the nail.

10. **IF**: Index Finger—tapping the edge point at the base of the nail.

11. **MF**: Middle Finger—tapping the edge point at the base of the nail.

12. **LF**: Little Finger—tapping the edge point at the base of the nail.

13. **KC**: Karate Chop point—side of the hand, where you would hit doing a karate chop.

14. **GP**: Gamut Point—tapping between the little finger and ring finger.

The Sequence

Using your fingertips for tapping, apply firm pressure of tap, tap, tapping on each of the points in sequence. If you have long fingernails, use the pads of your fingers to apply the tapping pressure.

Tapping should be firm but not too hard as to hurt or cause injury. It can be done on either side of the body as the points are bilateral. Use whichever side feels most comfortable — or you can swap from side to side.

1. Start by repeating the setup phrase three times while rubbing the sore spot (**SS**).
2. Repeat the reminder phrase while tapping with 2 or 3 fingers about 7 times on each of the other points.
3. Start at the eyebrow (**EB**) point and work down finishing at the karate chop point (**KC**) (disregarding the gamut point **GP**.)
4. To finish, repeat the setup phrase while tapping the karate chop point (**KC**), and include a phrase that allows you to let go of the pain and/or forgive those who may have been involved.

An example may be...

"Even though I am angry at Ellen for what she did this morning, I deeply and completely love and accept myself. I choose to forgive her for what she has done."

Nine-step Gamut Procedure

This is perhaps one of the strangest of all parts in EFT. It is basically a brain balancing exercise which has the added affect of cutting through mental or emotional conflict.

The Nine-step Gamut procedure is immediately followed by the EFT sequence. There are 9 steps to the sequence which are all carried out while tapping the Gamut Point (**GP**) and remaining focused on the problem. They are…

1. Shut your eyes
2. Open your eyes
3. Look hard down right
4. Look hard down left
5. Roll your eyes around clockwise
6. Roll your eyes counter clockwise
7. Hum a tune for 5 seconds
8. Count to 5
9. Hum again for 5 seconds

While this may seem like complete nonsense, there is logic behind it. Your mind is connected to your eyes, and different parts correspond to different eye movements. This is perhaps most recognized in Neuro-Linguistic Programming (NLP).

By opening and closing your eyes and then moving them in different directions, various parts of your brain are activated.

Your brain works in two halves—the left and the right hemispheres. The left is associated with logic and counting, whilst the right side is more creative.

In the nine gamut sequence, we activate both hemispheres by humming and counting. This procedure is particularly useful when dealing with problems such as, dyslexia.

An EFT Session

1. Start by identifying the problem.
2. Identify your intensity level and then create a setup and reminder phrase.
3. Do the EFT sequence, followed by the nine-step gamut procedure.
4. Start again at the beginning of Step 1 with another sequence.

Once you have done a round or two, stop and close your eyes and re-evaluate your problem. Measure your intensity level.

If there is still some emotional intensity left, do another round. This time however, change the setup phrase to start with, *"even though I have this remaining..."*

So in the example of a headache, you would say...

> *"Even though I have this remaining headache, I deeply and completely love and accept myself."*

The reminder phrase should also be changed to *"this remaining..."*

Keep checking and repeating the steps until your problem has reached an intensity level of zero.

If after several rounds you are getting stuck, have a look at some of the basic troubleshooting ideas which are listed at the end of Part II.

A Session Summarized

- Identify the problem and/or the pain, and measure its intensity from 0–10.
- Create a setup and reminder phrase that feels right. Be specific.
- Repeat your setup phrase 3 times while rubbing the sore spot (**SS**).
- Repeat reminder phrase while tapping on each of the following points 7 times... **EB, SE, UE, UN, UL, CB, UA, TN, IF, MF** and **LF**.
- Repeat the setup phrase while tapping **KC**. Finish by forgiving and letting go.
- Do the nine-step gamut procedure (remember to keep tapping **GP**).
- Repeat the sequence.
- Check and identify your intensity level.
- Repeat if necessary with *"this remaining..."*
- Ensure the intensity level is down to a 0.
- Repeat and/or look at troubleshooting if necessary.

Stuck? Basic Troubleshooting

Sometimes you might not seem to be making any progress. If this is the case, one of the following may help:

- Try a different setup phrase. Ensure you are being as specific as possible.
- Drink a glass of water. This can help provide insight.
- Move around. Some gentle exercise may help shift whatever is stuck.
- Say the setup and reminder phrases with force, exaggerating the wording. Such as, *"this really, really terrible headache."*
- Persistence and patience is sometimes all that is needed.

Part III

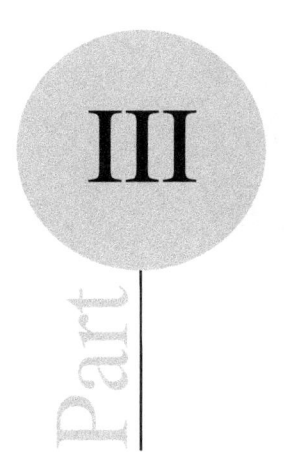

Advanced EFT Techniques

www.TheHiddenSecretsofEFT.com

Aspects: Layers Behind Layers

When working on a problem, there may be many different aspects or layers underlying the problem that emerge during the session. Each aspect needs to be treated separately.

You may find for example, treating a "fear of flying", you could simply say: *"this fear of flying"* and have total success.

More often though, you're likely to discover different aspects and layers behind the original problem that will need addressing before your fear of flying is completely resolved.

You may have fear of taking off, a fear of sitting next to someone you don't know, a fear of turbulence, a fear of being confined to a tiny space while using the aircraft toilet, or a fear of feeling trapped.

If different aspects do exist, each one must be identified and treated as a separate issue. It's best to begin on the most feared aspect, and then work your way backwards.

New fears may be identified or come up as you are treating something else. For example, if you are tapping on the fear of using the aircraft toilet, you may find you have a fear of walking there whilst airborne that is the root of the fear.

New fears (or root fears), often crop up. Go with whatever comes up for you. It may be useful to map out the different aspects. Remember to measure your intensity level before and after tapping.

www.TheHiddenSecretsofEFT.com

Treating the Abstract

Some people say that if you're not in the moment and experiencing the problem you are tapping for, then you are only treating an abstract concept. This is a valid comment.

Plus, you won't know if you are fully treated until you've come face to face with the problem again. Only then, will you know if EFT has dissolved all emotional intensity.

Obviously, some cases are harder to test than others.

In the case of "fear of flying", it is impractical and expensive to book a flight *just to see* if EFT has worked.

In cases such as these, experiencing the problem in your head and feeling if there is anxiety or not in your body, is proof whether progress has been made.

Other situations are easier to test; such as, fear of heights, public speaking or spiders. They're all examples of situations you can deliberately put yourself in to see if the fear has gone. A fun exercise to know for sure.

If you feel any remaining fear or anxiety, tap at the time to clear the emotional intensity.

Muscle Testing

Muscle testing has been an integral part of the original Thought Field Therapy (TFT) and other energy therapies. EFT however, eliminates the need for muscle testing by treating all points and any psychological reversal as standard.

That said, muscle testing is a useful skill to learn if you plan on using EFT as a tool to facilitate other people's healing. (And can improve your success rates enormously for specific problems, such as allergies.)

When you use muscle testing you can determine what areas someone tests "weak" for, and even test what could be the best potential treatment.

If you are not familiar with muscle testing, here is a brief guide. (I do however, recommend you learn from a more qualified source if you plan on using muscle testing on a regular basis.)

Have the person you are treating stand next to you with their arm outstretched, parallel to the floor. With their other hand, have them place it palm down on top of their head.

With the arm that's outstretched, ask them to hold their arm up while you apply a small amount of pressure on their wrist to test how strong the muscle feels. This is not a test of strength. It is only to feel the natural resistance in the deltoid muscle.

Now have them place the hand on their head, upside down with the back of the hand on top of their head. Apply pressure, and test the outstretched arm again for any weakness.

You should be able to note a difference between the two. For some people the difference will be great, while for others it will be much more subtle. Practice is needed to get consistent reliable results.

www.TheHiddenSecretsofEFT.com

Next, have them drop their hand on top of the head and say, *"my name is (their name)"* and test again. Next say, *"my name is Mickey Mouse"* and test. Again, you should be able to discern a difference in strength, where the false statement causes the arm to test weak (i.e. the person may not be able to hold their arm up in the outstretched position).

Once you have calibrated yourself with your client, simply have them make a statement that you wish to check and test. If someone wants to lose weight and you have them say, *"I want to lose weight"* and they test weak, this is a sign of psychological reversal and must be treated with a well phrased setup statement.

If they hold a substance to their chest that you suspect as being a problem and they test weak, then this confirms your suspicions. Treat with EFT and test again, repeating until a strong response is achieved (i.e. the arm tests strong and stays up with applied pressure).

The most important thing with any of these tests is that you "get yourself out of the way", trust yourself and the process. That is, you do not influence the result by holding any expectations of the outcome.

If you do hold expectations, you may get a false result. For this reason it's easier testing someone else than yourself.

Additional Points

There are estimations of more than 1500 acupuncture points on the body. Luckily, only 14 are used with EFT. We tap on these 14 points for all issues. This is because in most cases more than one meridian is involved with any issue.

Some EFT Therapists have experimented and noted that using additional points can be useful, speeding up the time it takes to get to the root of a problem.

Below I have singled out four additional points that are commonly used. These additional points can be integrated as you feel best into your EFT sessions, but are not essential for most cases.

You may connect with a certain point and choose to include it with the other points in your regular tapping routine. Often this decision is intuitive and instinctual. You may find certain issues shift faster when you tap on these additional points.

Top of the Head

This point is found on the centre of the highest point of the head, directly between the tops of the two ears. This point is known as the Crown Chakra.

According to Traditional Chinese Medicine (TCM), tapping this point stimulates the yang meridians encouraging energy down to lower parts of the body. (The yang meridians include the large intestine, small intestine, stomach, bladder and gall bladder.)

In Ayurveda Medicine, stimulating this point regulates the vata dosha, which balances the mind and emotions.

Personally, I find this point to be powerful and effective. Whilst introducing a new and positive thought pattern, I encourage my clients to tap the top of their head.

Under the Nipple

This point is situated on the rib directly below the nipple about where the fold of the breast meets the chest wall on a woman. For a man, this point is located about three inches below the nipple.

(Many EFT Therapists use a point just below this, on the bottom fixed rib, as this lies on the same meridian but is less awkward in a clinic situation.)

This point corresponds to the liver meridian and is especially useful when anger issues are not shifting or when there is a build-up of excessive resentment. For myself, I've found this point useful in times of stress.

Under the Wrist

If you use your whole hand to pat the underpart of the wrist, you won't miss this point. Alternatively, you can cross one wrist over the other and tap the insides of your wrists together.

Just like tapping on the top of the head, tapping under the wrist can quickly bring balance to your system in emergency situations or at intense points during an EFT round.

Ankle Points

Just above the ankle on both the inside and outside of the lower shin is where these points are. So you don't miss it, pat this area with your whole hand.

Tapping the ankle points is contraindicated for pregnancy. If you plan on falling pregnant or are at any stage in your pregnancy, it may be harmful to tap on these points.

Acupuncturists do not use this point, and teachers of Qi Gong and Nei Gong strictly forbid it.

In TCM, tapping the ankle points stimulates the yin meridians, sending energy to the upper parts of the body. (The yin meridians include the lung, heart, spleen, kidney and liver.)

Shortcuts

Doing a complete round may seem simple enough, however you can make it shorter still.

The following suggestions have been developed by a range of EFT Therapists through practice, trial and error.

It is recommended that you first become fully familiar with the complete round before shortcutting, so you always know what to do when the abbreviated sequence does not work.

Many therapists are now leaving out the nine-step gamut procedure, using it only when little progress is being made. This makes no difference to the treatment, other than to reduce time (and to ease a sceptical mind).

www.TheHiddenSecretsofEFT.com

In most cases, going straight to the karate chop point after doing the face and body (and leaving out the points on the fingers), works just as well as the full sequence. (This will save you another 10 seconds!)

Some EFT Therapists prefer to keep these points in as they believe the treatment is more effective.

My advice is to experiment and see what works best for you. Trust your intuition with each case.

Using the karate chop point instead of the sore point for the setup phrase at the beginning of each round works most of the time. (This is easier for group and telephone work.) When doing this, you can also leave it out at the end of the sequence.

When a client is experiencing intense pain in the present moment, often the setup and reminder phrases can be dropped. The client's attention is already focused on the problem. This is also good to calm them down so you can start a full treatment.

If things are really bad, using just the karate chop point is useful to start with. Use only the points that seem to work best. Often you will find that a client will experience a shift on 1 or 2 specific points.

If this is the case, you can focus on just the point(s) that seem to be working most effectively. When your intuition is heightened, you will just "know" which points to tap on and which points you can leave out.

If the results you are hoping for are not being achieved while doing this, you can simply start again using the full sequence.

Energy Toxins

Sometimes EFT does not seem to work, or the results are only temporary. If you find this to be the case, the problem may lie in an energy toxin causing a disruption to the energy system.

An energy toxin is simply another name for an allergy or sensitivity.

If someone has an allergy or sensitivity, this can cause a disruption in the energy system which may interfere with any EFT progress or treatment.

(While not all sensitivities block EFT, this is a problem for 10% to 20% of people.)

If an energy toxin appears to be hindering the progress, it can be dealt with in two ways: avoid it or treat it.

One fairly common culprit is laundry powder. This can easily be tested by having the client take a shower without soap and then tap before getting dressed.

If they feel a difference, then use EFT to treat for a sensitivity to washing powder.

If progress is made in a session but then the problem suddenly comes back, look at what may have been eaten or what substances the client may have come into contact with. These too should then be tested and treated.

Story Technique

If you are using EFT to treat others, the Story Technique is a great tool for working through an issue without them being overwhelmed by their feelings. It's also useful to ensure all aspects of a trauma are treated.

When recounting a past event, have them start at the beginning. Ask them to give their story a title, and an approximate time frame in which it happened.

Ask them for an intensity level on just saying the title. Tap on this before they even begin telling the story.

Once they are at a zero, request they begin to tell their story. As soon as they feel any emotional intensity—stop. (It is important you remain observant to any visual or auditory clues of emotional stress.)

Treat whatever is happening at this point until their intensity level reaches a zero.

Next, have them repeat the story from the beginning, again stopping at the first signs of emotional stress. Keep doing this until the whole event can be recounted without an upset.

When they are recounting their whole story, often other memories will surface. These may need treating, either at the time or at a later date. It's important to progress at their own speed and respect their experience.

Stepping Stone Technique

Sometimes it may be necessary to take things slowly and in stages. Perhaps there has been a long-standing issue and your whole identity has been built around this issue.

If this is the case, working in small stages is a much better approach, than bulldozing straight in.

An example would be, treating for agoraphobia. First you would tap until you could walk comfortably to your front door. The next week, you would tap until you were able to open the door without feeling any anxiety.

Next, you would walk to the front gate, and then to the local shops, and eventually into town or local fields.

Baby steps are the key here. Time between sessions is by choice and what suits you best.

Non-directive Technique

This can be used for your own personal development; or when a person feels something doesn't feel right but can't quite put their finger on what the cause is.

Non-directive tapping is a generalized technique that "shakes loose" underlying issues that have not yet fully surfaced. You can use this technique to give your body a "tune up".

Start by using an open setup phrase such as this...

> "Even though I have this problem, I deeply and completely love and accept myself."

After one or two rounds of this, you should find issues or emotions beginning to surface. Treat each one specifically as they arise.

Keyword Technique

This can be used when either a reminder phrase becomes too long and awkward to use. You can also use the Keyword Technique when you are too distraught to think about your problem.

A keyword or short phrase is identified and substituted for the problem.

It can be relevant or completely disconnected to your issue. All that matters is that you link that keyword in your mind to your problem. Think of it as a code word.

When using a keyword approach, an example setup phrase would be…

> *"Even though I have this turnip problem, I deeply and completely love and accept myself."*

The reminder phrase would then also become *"this turnip problem"*. In this example, the "turnip" is replacing the word of whatever the actual problem may be.

If you are using EFT on someone else, the Keyword Technique is useful if they are too ashamed or hurt to talk about their problem.

If you are treating family or close friends, you don't need to know their problems. While it is not uncommon that once they have successfully dealt with an issue, they may feel comfortable to openly share their experience without shame or pain; however, this should not be forced.

Memory Retrieval

Another of EFT's amazing benefits is its ability to often find lost or hidden memories. This can be used for convenient circumstances; such as, *"I can't remember where I left my car keys"* or for therapeutic treatments.

In therapy, it is useful for finding why a pattern or emotion has been established. In this case you could use a phrase such as…

"Even though I don't know why I have this illness, I deeply and completely love and accept myself."

"Even though I don't remember who caused me this pain, I deeply and completely love and accept myself."

Sometimes the memory comes back instantly. Other times it may be delayed or memories triggered that lead to the desired outcome. Once the desired memory has surfaced, and you find it holds—then treat it.

Tearless Trauma Technique (TTT)

The *Tearless Trauma Technique* (TTT) was developed by Gary Craig to help those deal with traumatic events too intense to even think about.

Although TTT is very gentle, it is as effective as any other approach. As with EFT in general, its simplicity should not be overlooked.

Start by identifying the problem from a distance, making sure you don't even think about the problem yet.

Ask yourself what you think the intensity level might be if you were to visualize or feel the problem. Now treat this probable feeling with EFT in the standard way.

> *"Even though if I were to think about this event I would be very upset, I deeply and completely love and accept myself."*

Once you have reached a zero, begin to get closer in your mind to the problem or event.

As with the Story Approach, treat each step that brings up an intensity level. Do this until all stages are complete, you feel you can think about it, and you can also describe in vivid detail the event without any emotional intensity.

The Choices Method

Developed by Patricia Carrington (Ph.D.) called the *Choices Method* adds a new dimension to the setup phrase. It does just what it says—it gives the user a choice—a positive

www.TheHiddenSecretsofEFT.com

alternative to your current experience. Once EFT has removed the problem, a void can remain in which we can create a new positive perspective.

It is important that the choice be introduced when the current problem has begun to shift, so that the subconscious does not reject it instantly.

To give an example how this might work, let's take a sensitivity to dairy products. We might use a setup phrase and choice such as this…

> *"Even though I have a problem with dairy products, I deeply and completely love and accept myself. I now choose to allow my body to be in harmony with all dairy products."*

If the choice was presented straight away, your subconscious may still view dairy products as a threat. So the idea of living in harmony with it may be rejected immediately.

To avoid this, start with 2 or 3 rounds of EFT without the choice, then any psychological reversal will be corrected. The disruption in your energy system causing the sensitivity will be cleared or reduced.

Now your choice will be easily accepted. Follow this sequence for the *Choices Method*…

1. Do a round of straight EFT without any choice.

2. Follow this with a sequence of tapping—just stating the choice as the reminder phrase, followed by a sequence of alternating the reminder phrase with the choice on each of the points.

3. Ensure you finish on a positive choice. If the last point is the standard reminder phrase then add an extra point, perhaps on the top of the head.

Borrowing Benefits

Developed from observations at many seminars, Borrowing Benefits is ideal for group work, where many people can be "helped" at once.

Everyone in the group identifies a personal issue and gives it a Subjective Unit of Distress (SUD) rating between 0-10.

One member of the group is then chosen, and the group leader takes them through the tapping process while everyone else joins in, tapping for that individual.

Once the person being worked on reaches a zero, everyone else in the group revisits their problem and checks their intensity.

Interestingly most people in the group will now be at a very low or completely clear level (therapists report between 70% to 100% of group members experience this).

Then, another person is chosen with a remaining issue and the group works on them until they are clear. This keeps happening until everyone has cleared their issue.

It is useful to note, that not everyone needs to be working on the same issue or even the same type of problem. You could have some people work on physical pain while others are working on addictions or emotional abuse.

It is important to have other trained EFT Therapists on hand to keep an eye out for any members in the group who may become overwhelmed. (They may need to be taken aside for individual attention.)

Double Crossed Hand Technique

EFT has traditionally been taught to be applied on one side of the body, or even tapping both sides and sometimes both hands.

More recently it has been suggested that tapping be done using both hands crossed over, tapping on the opposite side of your body.

This can be a little tricky for some of the points, but in my experience, it does seem to speed up the treatment. (It seems particularly effective when there is a conflict or paradox in the client's emotions or thinking.)

The crossing of the hands has been used by several therapies now including the cross crawl and hook ups found in Brain Gym™ exercises, and seems to integrate well with EFT.

As with any EFT variation, experiment and trust your intuition when deciding the best approach.

Eyes to Ceiling Technique

This is a simplified version of the Nine-step Gamut Procedure and is best used to clear a remaining 1–2 level of intensity.

While you tap the gamut spot, look at your hand so you look down as far as possible, keeping your head straight at all times.

Raise your hand, taking 6–8 seconds, and watch it as you raise your hand as high as possible.

Then lower your hand back down to the floor, watching with your eyes. As you watch your hand being lowered, give yourself permission to let go of your problem.

(This usually saves time, by eliminating the need to repeat a full sequence.)

During this whole procedure you should remain focused as much as possible on the problem. Think about your reminder phrase to keep focused.

Touch and Breath (TAB)

Touch and Breath (TAB), was developed by Dr. John Diepold Jr. Ph.D.

In this technique, you touch the acupressure point lightly and take a deep breath while focusing on your problem.

This technique illustrates that tapping is not always necessary.

EFT tapping and pressure may feel uncomfortable, may have restricted movement and/or may be difficult to do in a public place. TAB is a great alternative.

Clients Without Emotion

Some clients may feel disconnected from their emotions and unable to give an intensity level for a specific problem—even for events that would typically have a high emotional charge.

In this situation, the Validity of Cognition (VOC) scale comes in handy.

VOC is similar to the 0–10 SUD level, except it is a measure of how true something is to yourself or the client.

Initially the problem that's being tapped on may feel very true, and ranked at a 9 or 10 intensity level. After a few rounds of tapping, a cognitive shift may occur, allowing the client to see that the problem is now less true or even invalid.

To avoid problems like the Apex Effect, it's suggested the client record their sessions and measure their intensity levels like the SUD method. This will enable the client to observe how much progress they're making from one session to the next.

VOC can be used to observe past events, describe problems related to a scene—looking at how clear the imagery and sounds are, and identifying the affect on one's life.

Measure a VOC between 0–10, then tap. Notice any change as more rounds of tapping take place. If or when your emotions return, you can switch back to the SUD method.

Key Questions

To get to the root of a problem or find the core issue, some important key questions can be asked. Many of the answers may surprise you.

It's not necessary to ask these questions for every session, but is useful to stimulate your own line of enquiry and trigger your thought processes.

Some useful examples are given below…

- When did this first start?
- What happened around this time?
- What are you most angry at?
- What in your life do you wish most had never happened?
- What is the most traumatic thing that has ever happened to you?
- If you did not have this problem, what else would you be doing or what may happen?
- How does this problem serve you?
- Are you ready to let go of this problem?
- Who do you most blame and why?
- What and/or who are you most afraid of?
- What do you want most in life? Why don't you have it?

- What is the major reoccurring pattern in your life?
- What do you most dislike about yourself?

Once you have clearly identified some answers, you can commence your EFT session using many of the techniques described in this chapter.

www.TheHiddenSecretsofEFT.com

Part IV

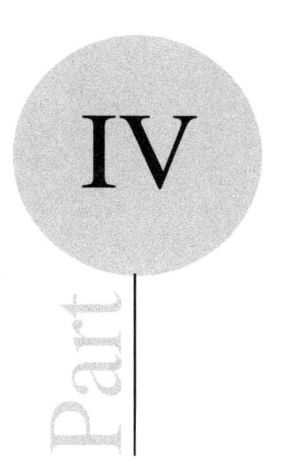

The Hidden Secrets of EFT

www.TheHiddenSecretsofEFT.com

Skyrocket Your Self-esteem

"You yourself, as much as anybody in the entire universe, deserves your love and affection."
~ **Buddha**

Do You Love Yourself?

Fact: Most of us have low self-esteem; however, I'm about to demonstrate how to greatly increase it using EFT.

It may be generalizing to say, but I believe to some degree we all suffer from low self-esteem—and that we could all do with a healthy boost.

Addressing our own levels of self-esteem first, will help address all other future problems when using EFT.

The setup phrase of EFT uses: *"I deeply and completely love myself,"* yet how many of us can honestly say we do?

Let's address the love part first and then we'll move onto acceptance.

Tell yourself aloud that you love yourself, and then listen to the self-talk that immediately comes to the surface.

Perhaps you automatically think, "No I don't." Perhaps you think you're not smart enough, not good enough, or not deserving enough. Whatever you may think, perhaps in some way you believe you are "not enough."

Whatever first comes up for you is what you need to tap on and address first. Here are some examples…

> *"Even though I don't love myself, I deeply and completely love and accept myself anyway. I now choose to be open to loving myself more."*
>
> *"Even though I am not worthy of my own love, I deeply and completely love and accept myself anyway. I now choose to*

be open to loving myself more."

"Even though I am not good enough, I deeply and completely love and accept myself anyway. I now choose to be open to loving myself more."

"Even though I am not smart enough, I deeply and completely love and accept myself anyway. I now choose to be open to loving myself more."

"Even though I am not good-looking enough, I deeply and completely love and accept myself anyway. I now choose to be open to loving myself more."

"Even though I am not enough, I deeply and completely love and accept myself anyway. I now choose to be open to loving myself more."

"Even though I am not perfect and cannot possibly love myself, I deeply and completely love and accept myself anyway. I now choose to be open to loving myself more."

Keep tapping until your intensity level is at a zero. If you find yourself going off on a tangent, write it down and address it another time.

If you find you don't know why you don't like yourself, you can tap on the setup phrase below. Tap on whatever comes up for you...

"Even though I don't love myself and I don't know why, I deeply and completely love and accept myself anyway. I now choose to be open to loving myself more."

It may be that you only love parts of yourself and not all of yourself. If this is true for you, then tap on loving all of yourself...

> *"Even though I only love some parts of myself and not my whole self, I deeply and completely love and accept myself anyway. I now choose to be open to loving myself more."*
>
> *"Even though only some aspects of me deserve to be loved and there are some parts of myself I despise, I deeply and completely love and accept myself anyway. I now choose to be open to loving myself more."*

Do You Accept Yourself?

The other part of the main EFT setup phrase is: *"I deeply and completely accept myself."*

Just like many can't say we love ourselves, not many of us can truly say we accept ourselves.

Tell yourself aloud that you accept yourself. And then, just like you did previously, listen to what self-talk immediately comes up for you.

Perhaps you automatically think, "No I don't." Perhaps you wish you could accept yourself but don't know how. Perhaps you are tougher on yourself than on anyone else you know.

Perhaps you think it is conceited, or high and mighty to completely accept yourself.

Whatever pops into your mind first, is what you need to address. Turn your objections into setup phrases. Address the objections that first come into your head. Here are some examples...

> "Even though I don't accept myself, I deeply and completely love and accept myself anyway. I now choose to be open to accepting myself more each day."

> "Even though I want to accept myself, but I don't know how, I deeply and completely love and accept myself anyway. I now choose to be open to accepting myself more each day."

> "Even though I accept others but I refuse to accept myself, I deeply and completely love and accept myself anyway. I now choose to be open to accepting myself more each day."

> "Even though I believe it is conceited and stuck up to accept myself, I deeply and completely love and accept myself anyway. I now choose to be open to accepting myself more each day."

If you find you don't know why you don't accept yourself, you can tap on this setup phrase below...

> "Even though I don't accept myself and I don't know why, I deeply and completely love and accept myself anyway. I now choose to be open to accepting myself more each day."

It may also be that you only accept certain parts of yourself and not all of yourself. If this is true for you, then tap on accepting all of yourself...

> "Even though I can only accept some parts of myself, and not my whole self, I deeply and completely love and accept

myself anyway. I now choose to be open to accepting myself more each day."

"Even though only some aspects of me deserve to be accepted, and there are some parts of me I hate, I deeply and completely love and accept myself anyway. I now choose to be open to accepting myself more each day."

"Even though I can only accept myself once I am perfect (and I'll never be perfect and therefore never accept myself), I deeply and completely love and accept myself anyway. I now choose to be open to accepting myself more."

What Do Others Think of Me?

Perhaps you pay more attention to what others think of you and how they perceive you, rather than how you perceive yourself.

If this is the case, you are bound to suffer from low self-esteem. While it is dangerous to take on other's opinions and beliefs about you as your own, it is also a natural thing to do — especially when you're very young and impressionable.

It's time to change how you think of yourself, so you can view yourself through your own eyes. Loving and accepting yourself becomes easier when you put yourself first, and are not constantly worrying and obsessing about what others think of you.

Here are some useful setup phrases so you can start putting yourself first...

"Even though I pay more attention to what others think of me than what I think of myself, I deeply and completely love and accept myself. I now choose to put myself first."

"Even though I find it high and mighty to put myself first—I was always taught to think of others first, I deeply and completely love and accept myself. I now choose to let go of this old belief as it no longer serves me."

"Even though I was taught to respect and believe what older people told me no matter what, I deeply and completely love and accept myself. I now choose to carefully examine what people say before accepting it as true."

"Even though society told me to listen to my parents, teachers and other people who knew better than me, I deeply and completely love and accept myself. I now choose to listen to myself first."

"Even though I have taken on what others have said about me as the absolute truth, I deeply and completely love and accept myself. I now choose to accept only the beliefs that help me, and to reject the rest."

Undoing Your Childhood Conditioning

From the time you were a baby, the attitudes and beliefs of those closest to you, would have impacted your life today.

When you were young, your unconditional love for the key people in your life; such as your parents, probably affected you and your beliefs in some way. This is because you would have believed everything they told you about yourself and took their beliefs on as absolute truth.

Now that you're older and wiser, you're in a position to let go of any beliefs you have adopted, that don't serve you today.

It wasn't just what you were told; it was also what had been modelled to you while you were young.

Often the behaviors you observed as a child, you would have unconsciously taken on-board as your own. No doubt there would have been some useful beliefs; however, there would have been many beliefs that have hindered you today.

EFT can help free you from these limiting beliefs.

Think back over your childhood and list all the limiting phrases that were repeated to you about love and acceptance. Then turn them into setup phrases. Here are some ideas to get you started...

> "Even though I was criticized or judged unfairly, I deeply and completely love and accept myself. I now choose to separate other's opinions of me as belonging to them and not me."

> "Even though I felt rejected and unloved as a child, I deeply and completely love and accept myself. I now choose to validate myself and not rely on others."

> "Even though I made a terrible mistake in the past which I cannot forget, I deeply and completely love and accept myself. I now choose to lay the past at rest and focus on the present moment."

www.TheHiddenSecretsofEFT.com

> *"Even though I was laughed at as a child and felt I was no good, I deeply and completely love and accept myself. I now choose to create a new reality in this moment now."*
>
> *"Even though I felt disappointed when _____ happened, I deeply and completely love and accept myself. I now choose to take the lesson from that experience and turn it into a positive."*

I Resent Other People and Their Life

Have you noticed that the few people who possess real self confidence are life's cheerleaders? They notice, appreciate and celebrate other's good. They tend to not grumble or complain when something great happens to others.

If you find it difficult to be happy for others, you may find the following setup phrases useful...

> *"Even though I resent so much... (other's personal qualities, belongings, relationships and other's opportunities), I deeply and completely love and accept myself. I now choose to be happy for the great things that happen to others and know that as I focus on their good, great things will come to me too."*
>
> *"Even though I am incapable of feeling happy for others as I deserve it more than they do, I deeply and completely love and accept myself. I now choose to be open to celebrating other's good."*

"Even though good stuff happens to everyone else but me and I feel left out, I deeply and completely love and accept myself. I now choose to believe good things can happen to me too if I allow it."

"Even though I feel bitter when other people's lives seem greater than mine, I deeply and completely love and accept myself. I choose to remember my first bitter experience and dissolve negativity around that."

"Even though I secretly feel happy when bad things happen to others, I deeply and completely love and accept myself. I choose to accept that like attracts like. And as long as I feel smug in the face of other's misfortune I can never experience peace inside myself."

I Feel Socially Awkward

You may feel socially awkward around other people and to some degree this is perfectly normal. Whether it's a feeling of apprehension at a large social gathering, meeting new people for the first time, or asking for help from somebody, EFT can help.

If you would like to exude more self-esteem, try these...

"Even though I am jealous of those who are at ease in social situations, I deeply and completely love and accept myself. I now choose to accept I can slowly change who I am, allowing myself to become more confident each day."

"Even though I feel I must compete and compare myself with others in social situations, I deeply and completely love and accept myself. I now choose to accept myself more, and in doing so, I am more accepting of others."

"Even though I feel tongue-tied in certain situations, I deeply and completely love and accept myself. I choose to acknowledge myself by speaking up, even if I feel uncomfortable at first."

"Even though I feel small and insignificant compared to certain others, I deeply and completely love and accept myself. I choose to accept that no one is better than anybody else, we are all one."

"Even though I wish I was more like X, I deeply and completely love and accept myself. I choose to use X as someone positive I can model, and consciously integrate the positive attributes I admire so much, into me."

I Postpone My Happiness

Perhaps you don't feel you can be happy in the present moment, until you have achieved something in the future. Those with healthy and high self-esteem accept themselves no matter where they are.

Tap on these to free yourself from living in the future...

"Even though I cannot possible be happy until I have done _____, I deeply and completely love and accept myself. I now choose to be happy no matter what."

"Even though I'm being unrealistic about what I can achieve and I'm applying undue pressure on myself, I deeply and completely love and accept myself. I now choose to set myself up for success by choosing achievable goals."

"Even though I can only be happy when... (I've found true love, I've gotten married, I've had children, I've bought a house, I've got this job, I've got this much money, I've achieved my ideal weight), I deeply and completely love and accept myself. I choose to accept that by living in the future, I am preventing myself from enjoying now."

"Even though it is natural for me to postpone happiness and I don't know how to break this habit, I deeply and completely love and accept myself. I choose to uncover the root of why I cannot live now."

"Even though I do not know how to be happy in this moment right here and now, I deeply and completely love and accept myself. I now choose to embrace and be more aware of each present moment."

I Wish I Had More Confidence

Those people with that quiet air of confidence take full responsibility for their lives (good and bad). They do not blame others, and are not afraid to stand up for what they believe in.

Use these setup phrases to increase your charisma...

"Even though I don't want to take full responsibility for my life, I deeply and completely love and accept myself. I now choose to accept I am the only one who can live my life. No one else can live it for me."

"Even though I blame X for doing _____, I deeply and completely love and accept myself. I now choose to accept others exactly as they are, warts and all."

"Even though I do not listen to my heart, I deeply and completely love and accept myself. I now choose to listen to my inner voice more every day."

"Even though I am too scared to stand up for what I believe in, I deeply and completely love and accept myself. I now choose to live my beliefs quietly through my actions without forcing what I believe onto anyone else."

"Even though I crave the validation of others before I can validate myself, I deeply and completely love and accept myself. I choose to validate me and put myself first. It isn't anyone else's responsibility but mine!"

As You Change, Others Around You Will Change Too

As your self-esteem increases and your behavior changes accordingly, you will notice a change in others. It's a natural progression that when you truly love and accept yourself, others will too.

Be aware that when you are tapping on one thing, something else will likely come up. Effectively a can of worms can be opened and it may require many sessions to clear all your self-esteem issues.

Know that finding the root issues are usually causing a host of other smaller issues. When you dissolve these root issues, you'll find you won't need to tap on many others as they won't be relevant any more.

With each issue that you tap away, be encouraged that your self-esteem is growing from strength to strength.

Do not be in a hurry to "tap out everything" in a short time. You don't want to overload yourself. Keep persisting.

Be sure you completely clear one issue entirely before moving onto the next.

Case Study

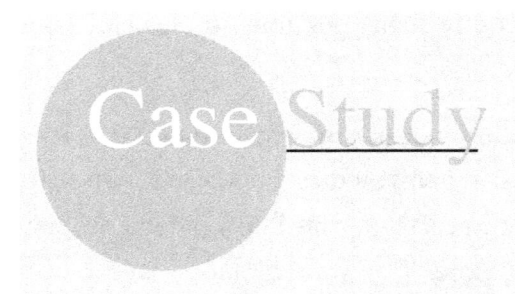

One EFT client that I worked with, would constantly compare himself to others, never felt good enough, nor was able to trust his own judgement.

It seemed as though he always attracted situations in his life where he was criticized, and that left him feeling unsure of himself. All of these experiences and reactions were connected to low self-esteem.

We started by tapping on particular interactions that occurred at work with his boss…

> *"Even though my boss criticized me and made me feel terrible, maybe I can choose to let that go and love and accept myself anyway, knowing I did my best."*
>
> *"Even though my boss told me that my work was not good enough and that I didn't do the job properly, I love and accept myself anyway and now choose to feel calm and confident instead."*

When I asked my client: "What did this feeling remind him of," he was then able to recall another situation with a coworker that criticized him as well.

So we tapped on…

"Even though my coworker called me an idiot and made me feel terrible, I choose now to let that go and see the situation in a different light."

After clearing a few more similar situations at work we then began to move a little deeper into the process. He explained that he has never felt good enough when comparing himself to others.

We then tapped on the following statements…

"Even though I never feel good enough when I compare myself to others, maybe I can choose to let that go and begin to see all the positive qualities that I do have."

"Even though I never feel good enough compared to my coworkers, I now choose to accept myself anyway and recognize all my strengths instead."

"Even though I feel unsure about myself around my coworkers, I now choose to let that go and begin to feel confident and assured instead."

"Even though I feel unsure of my own decisions when my boss criticizes me, I now choose to love and accept myself anyway and feel confident in myself instead."

At this point, I asked my client: "What was the earliest memory of this same feeling," and "What did the feeling remind him of?" This would help identify the root or starting point of the issue.

My client was able to say that he had a teacher that always made him feel unsure of his decisions and that his mom criticized his choices as well. This led to tapping on the statements below…

> *"Even though I felt stupid in front of the class when my teacher, Mrs. Smith, asked me a question I couldn't answer, maybe I can choose to that let go and see the situation differently."*
>
> *"Even though I felt unsure of myself and my decisions when my teacher, Mrs. Smith, criticized me, I now choose to love and accept myself anyway, and feel confident in my abilities and choices instead."*
>
> *"Even though my mother criticized my choices about my career in front of dad, maybe I can choose to let that go and see the situation differently."*
>
> *"Even though I felt unsure of myself when my mother criticized me, I now choose to love and accept myself anyway, and trust my decisions and choices."*

Finally, I encouraged my client to identify any other situation or events that created a similar feeling of being criticized or unsure of himself in order to cover all "aspects".

My client was able to think of another event from his childhood with his sister that created that same feeling.

We tapped on the following…

> *"Even though my sister told me that I was doing it wrong and*

I should do it differently, I love and accept myself anyway. I now choose to see that situation in a more loving light."

"Even though my sister criticized me and I felt like I could not trust myself and my decisions, I love and accept myself anyway and now choose to feel the decisions I make for me are the right ones."

At this time, when I asked my client to reflect back on making decisions at work and trusting himself, he was able to feel that he could do so with 100% confidence.

Low self-esteem often has multiple aspects to it, so I gave him a "tapping script" for everyday use to continue to improve his overall self-esteem.

This was the tapping script given to the client…

"Even though I had this low self-esteem because others criticized my choices and decisions, I love and accept myself anyway, fully and completely. I now choose to feel confident and sure of my decisions instead."

I recommended that he tap everyday on the above statement for 5 minutes in the morning, 5 minutes before bed; as well as tapping on any other aspects that may come up over the next days.

After checking in with my client two months later he reported that his self-esteem had increased dramatically and that he had never felt so good about himself or confident in years!

www.TheHiddenSecretsofEFT.com

Free Yourself From Fear and Anxiety For Good

"You gain strength, courage, and confidence by every experience in which you really stop to look fear in the face. You must do the thing which you think you cannot do."
~ Eleanor Roosevelt

7 Types of Fear

Fear is a primal emotional response to anything that we perceive as a threat to our safety. We all experience fear to varying degrees in our lives.

Fear is a normal human emotion that is temporarily experienced at the time of the perceived or real threat. And because the emotion of fear is so complex, it's likely you may experience different levels of fear on a regular basis.

Through practising EFT, I have identified 7 types of fear. Let's take a closer look at each one in detail...

1. Real Fear

When an incident happens that you perceive as being threatening or dangerous to your survival, your primal "fight or flight" instinct kicks in. This is called Real Fear.

A friend of mine once told me his story that illustrates real fear perfectly which he has allowed me to share...

A few years ago, he was visiting Chitwan National Park in Nepal and was on a guided walk. His guide warned him that if he ever saw a rhino, that he was to run in zigzag lines and then climb up the nearest tree.

During his guided walk, my friend was lucky enough to see a sleeping mother rhino with her baby.

Suddenly his guide ran towards him and screamed at him to run!

My friend recalls not remembering much about running in zigzag lines or scrambling up a tree. He recalls his real fear kicking in after he was "safely" up his tree.

He said his adrenaline took over at the time of danger. There was no time to feel any fear as his only thought was of survival.

2. Protective Fear

Protective fear is the logical thought processes that keep us out of danger. A lot can be put down to plain common sense and understanding our own limitations.

Protective fear is generally experienced because of a certain set of circumstances that present themselves to us which force us to make certain decisions.

Most of us would not drive a plane if we had no pilot's license or training. We wouldn't do this because we know we'd kill ourselves.

There are some people however, who do not listen to their common sense, and put themselves and others, in unnecessary danger.

3. Artificial Fear

Artificial fear is brought on by outside influences that change your body's chemistry. Living in an unhealthy environment — such as, in a busy city with too much electromagnetic pollution — can create anxiety in your body.

Too many "time saving" gadgets emit harmful radiation, and can cause ill-health, anxiety and fear.

Obviously, the best thing to do is avoid the cause; however, for many of us it's impractical to move to the country, or stop using all electrical devices.

The next best thing is to take regular breaks from your unhealthy living environment—get away every weekend if you can. Enjoy breathing fresh, clean air, and feel your accumulated anxiety lessen as your batteries are literally recharged.

While you may not be able to choose where you live, you *can* change your lifestyle choices. Smoking, over-consumption of alcohol, and/or using prescriptive/recreational drugs can also lead to various emotional and physiological imbalances.

4. Biophysical Fear

Many of us have bad body posture. In fact, when we see someone with "good posture" it is very noticeable because it is so rare.

The result of bad posture causes us to breath in a shallow way. This is unhealthy for us as it causes hyperventilation. Hyperventilation can cause anxiety, that can then lead to debilitating panic attacks.

Breathing properly is an art, one that we don't take seriously enough. Musicians who play wind instruments and trained singers, are taught how to breathe correctly.

The best way to breathe correctly is when you inhale your diaphragm and stomach should inflate, and when you exhale your diaphragm and stomach should deflate.

Practice this lying flat on the floor with a book on your stomach. This will show you when you're breathing correctly. Yoga and other similar training, can also teach correct breathing methods.

Whilst breathing seems to be a simple concept, the importance of breathing correctly cannot be overstated. It will reduce your anxiety, allowing you to experience a calm and peaceful state.

5. Illusionary or Learned Fears and Phobias

We all live with a range of fears, some so small that they have little or no impact on our lives, and others so great that they can develop into a phobia.

Some fears are learnt behaviors; for instance, we may take on the same fears and phobias our parents had in their lives. The terror or panic they experienced in certain circumstances may have been absorbed by us.

Like fear, phobias may have developed from a trauma or circumstance that occurred in our life when we were a child. Perhaps we were bitten by a dog, stung by a bee or fell out of a tree house.

Phobias often act as a debilitating hindrance in our lives. They may seem like a simple fear, but the irrational fear or phobia becomes more damaging than the actual problem that is causing the fear.

6. Intuitional Fear

We all have a natural awareness to positive or negative energy, and often notice people we dislike instinctively or feel may harm us.

Even in the animal world, intuition is strongly listened to. When an animal senses danger is approaching they will run away.

Intuitional fear is similar to protective fear—it can alert us to something in our environment or within our body that is wrong or imbalanced, and can act as a very helpful warning signal.

This guiding sense is experienced as a strong emotional feeling—many of us choose to ignore it. Instead of listening to our own instincts about self healing, we turn to others for help.

Learning to identify the anxiety that we feel when our intuition is alerting us to something being wrong, is the key to using this sense to our own advantage.

7. Growth Fear

Many of us experience discomfort when we are in new or unfamiliar situations. This discomfort can be experienced as apprehension or anxiety.

We must be clear that it is not the event itself that is causing us to feel uncomfortable, it is what we think will happen during that event that causes us the discomfort and anxiety.

Two factors will determine how uncomfortable we feel: 1. what we believe and 2. what we have experienced in the past. As the new situation becomes familiar to us and we recover our previous feelings, our anxiety usually fades.

Many successful people use these feelings of anxiety as a driving force to aim for something higher. They take themselves out of their comfort zones and relish the challenges these new opportunities and experiences bring them.

By accepting we'll feel uncomfortable with the unfamiliar and taking action despite our discomfort, we'll be able to achieve so much more in our lives.

Tips for Dispelling Fears

Now that you're aware of the different types of fears, it's time to work on tapping away your own fears. Although it's not essential, see if you can pin-point when you first felt your fear.

Approach your fear slowly, taking it in stages. As you think about and visualize your fear, measure your intensity level. If your fear is too overwhelming, take it down in stages whilst tapping down the emotional intensity until you can get closer to the actual fear.

Fear of the Unknown

Sometimes we live our lives in fear of the future. This stems from fear of not knowing and trusting the outcome to a situation, opportunity or experience. The only constant in life is change, so we can never know for sure what is around the corner.

What is certain though, that if we hide away in fear, we will limit living our life to its full potential.

Here are some setup phrases to help overcome these fears...

"Even though I am scared to live today because I don't know what will happen in the future, I deeply and completely love and accept myself. I choose to have the courage to live fully and trust I can cope with the outcome no matter what."

"Even though I don't know what my future holds, I deeply and completely love and accept myself. I choose to accept that no matter what happens, I am safe."

"Even though I am suspicious and wary of new people, situations or experiences, I deeply and completely love and accept myself. I choose to trust that every person, situation and experience in my life now, are in their perfect place."

"Even though I am frightened to attempt something different, I deeply and completely love and accept myself. I choose to feel comfortable with being uncomfortable, until my new comfort zone adjusts."

"Even though my fear of the future paralyzes me in living today, I deeply and completely love and accept myself. I

www.TheHiddenSecretsofEFT.com

choose to live fully each day, knowing it is OK to feel scared sometimes."

Fear of the Past

Perhaps something happened in your past that is stopping you from moving on with your life today. If you continue to hold onto limiting beliefs that no longer serve you today, you will suffer unnecessarily.

Please turn the fear of the past into a setup phrase, then choose how you would like to feel and have that as your choice at the end of the setup phrase.

You can use these as inspiration to get you started...

> "Even though I nearly drowned in the school swimming pool when I was 10 and I can't go near water now, I deeply and completely love and accept myself. I choose to forgive myself and all involved and to take small steps now to entering the water confidently."

> "Even though my teacher screamed at me for not doing it right and I've been scared of making any mistakes since, I deeply and completely love and accept myself. I choose to accept it is OK to make mistakes and to not be so hard on myself."

> "Even though my brother locked me in a dark closet when I was young and I'm petrified of small spaces now, I deeply and completely love and accept myself. I choose to try EFT to reduce my fear and anxiety."

Fear of Others

Often we pay more attention to what others think, say and do than we do ourselves. While it is useful to gain constructive feedback from others, it is not helpful to put other's opinions of ourselves ahead of our own.

Putting others before ourselves may have been instilled in us from an early age. Often we were taught that our parents and teachers knew better than us.

While this may have been the case when we were very young to protect us against ourselves, it may not be the case now.

Use the following setup phrases to encourage you to put yourself first...

> "Even though my mother and father always knew best and had the last word, I deeply and completely love and accept myself. I choose to understand I am old enough to know what is best for me now."

> "Even though I was not listened to because I was young, I deeply and completely love and accept myself. I choose to trust my voice is valid and to speak up when I have something to say."

> "Even though I don't feel good or worthy enough and think everyone else is better than me, I deeply and completely love and accept myself. I choose to see myself as an equal and as good as everyone else."

www.TheHiddenSecretsofEFT.com

"Even though I don't know how to act in social situations because others may reject me, I deeply and completely love and accept myself. I choose to understand that everyone is in the same boat and feels the same way."

"Even though I'm angry that my past has limited my actions and affected my choices today, I deeply and completely love and accept myself. I choose to act freely now creating a new past today."

Anxiety

Anxiety is different from fear and should therefore be addressed differently. Anxiety usually occurs without a threat from any external source.

Anxiety is becoming more common. If you suffer from anxiety, you may find yourself withdrawing from daily life. Even a trip to the local grocery store or picking up the children from school can seem like a struggle.

Because others around you cannot "see" what you are suffering from, it can make it all the more isolating.

A full blown anxiety or panic attack can be extremely frightening. Many people who have experienced a panic attack have reported thinking they were going to die, or were having a heart attack.

Physical symptoms such as palpitations, come on because of hyperventilation (basically fast, shallow breathing).

Hyperventilation causes other problems such as blurred vision, pins and needles and fainting.

Think about what triggers your anxiety and tune into how you feel, then phrase your setup statement accordingly. Here are some examples...

"Even though when I'm in a _____ situation I feel I can't even breathe, I deeply and completely love and accept myself. I choose to feel safe when I am in that _____ situation."

"Even though my chest tightens and I feel like I'm going to faint when _____, I deeply and completely love and accept myself. I choose to use EFT as soon as these physical symptoms present themselves."

"Even though I feel isolated, embarrassed and alone because no one understands what I'm going through, I deeply and completely love and accept myself. I choose to understand everyone has their own problems and may feel just like me."

"Even though I'm angry that my anxiety keeps me from participating fully in my everyday life, I deeply and completely love and accept myself. I choose to allow EFT to lower my emotional intensity, so I can actively take part in my life each day."

Panic Attacks and Feeling Out of Control

Experiencing anxiety can feel overwhelming. You may feel as if you are slowly sinking or drowning.

Perhaps the trigger to your anxiety may be so deeply hidden, a panic attack or heart palpitation can seemingly come from nowhere. Even a fleeting thought may trigger huge anxiety and cause havoc inside your physical body.

Even if you only have one attack in your life, you can suffer from the fear of having an attack on a daily basis. If you've had an anxiety attack before, the fear of having another attack can be enough to onset further attacks.

Through EFT, you may discover the trigger that causes your feelings of panic. It may be surprising what you find your trigger to be, as it may be something completely unrelated.

Regular practice of EFT will eradicate many physical symptoms of a panic attack, reducing your heart rate, slowing your breathing and feeling more relaxed.

If you have always lived in a mild state of anxiety it will feel extremely enjoyable to feel so calm. You may even feel sleepy.

Think about what scares you most about your panic attacks and turn them into setup phrases. Here are some examples...

"Even though I think about when, where and what might happen if I were to have another panic attack I deeply and completely love and accept myself. I choose to focus on the present moment and not worry myself over something that may never happen again."

"Even though I have a racing heart and difficulty breathing when I think about a potential panic attack, I deeply and completely love and accept myself. I now choose to be in control of this. I choose to act freely today, creating a new past today."

"Even though I am scared to lose control, I deeply and completely love and accept myself. I choose to trust my body to keep me safe at all times."

"Even though I feel helpless, alienated and misunderstood, I deeply and completely love and accept myself. I choose to confront the places, people and situations to feel in control of my anxiety."

Case Study

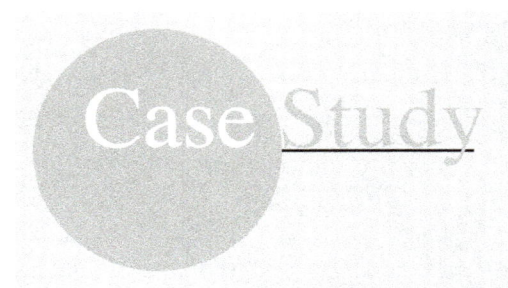

Fears and anxiety are often multilayered and complex so you may find some initial relief with just tapping on *"anxiety"*.

You will however, find greater success and more permanent relief if you're able to uncover all the different "aspects" and layers beneath your anxiety.

Below is a great example of a client who had anxiety and associated aspects, connected to an upcoming test.

The client had to do a test to upgrade her skills as an insurance agent at work. In order to pass the test, she had to receive a score of 70% or higher.

We began with a very general round of tapping before she was able to identify different aspects...

> *"Even though I have this anxiety about doing the test, I choose now to let it go and feel calm and confident instead."*

After bringing her anxiety number down a little, I asked her if she could identify specifically what she was worried about.

She stated she didn't know what building she was supposed to do the test in, and was afraid that if she couldn't find the building she'd be late or miss the test completely. So we tapped on…

> *"Even though I feel anxious about finding the building for my test tomorrow, I choose now to let that go and trust in myself and my sense of direction."*

Then she stated she was actually anxious about being late for her test more than any other reason, so we tapped on the following…

> *"Even though I feel anxious about my car breaking down tomorrow on the way to write my test, I now choose to let that feeling go and feel calm and confident instead, as I imagine myself arriving with ease."*

We also tapped on…

> *"Even though I still feel anxious about being late for my test tomorrow, I choose now to let that anxious feeling go and instead feel calm and relaxed as I imagine myself arriving on time."*

As she began to feel better about arriving at the right place at the right time to do her test, she then felt anxious about other things that could possibly go wrong.

We continued to tap on…

> *"Even though I feel anxious about the fact that my pen could run out of ink during the test and I won't be able to finish*

writing, I now choose instead to allow my mind to feel relaxed and open to a solution."

And then we tapped on…

"Even though I feel anxious about the fact that my pencil could break during the test and I won't be able to finish writing, I now choose instead to allow my mind to feel relaxed and open to a solution."

Once we had worked though those aspects, my client was able to identify more.

I asked her to actually imagine herself writing the test. We then tapped on…

"Even though I feel anxious because I could forget everything while writing the test, I love and accept myself anyway and now choose to let this anxious feeling go."

We also tapped on…

"Even though I feel anxious that I did not study enough for this test, I love and accept myself anyway and allow my mind to open up and recall all necessary information for this test."

And we also tapped on…

"Even though I'm afraid that I might freeze up during the test and not be able to write, I now choose to let that feeling go and feel calm, confident and relaxed instead."

I then asked my client to think about the "worse case scenario". For her, this was actually failing the test.

The reason for doing this, was for her to identify additional thoughts, fears, and "aspects" that needed to be cleared.

We then continued the tapping…

"Even though I'm really afraid that I will fail this test, I love and accept myself anyway, fully and completely. I now choose to let that fear go, knowing that I can deal with any outcome."

We also tapped on…

"Even though I'm afraid of what people will think if I fail the test, I love and accept myself anyway, and now choose to let go of caring about what other people might think."

We also discovered that she was feeling a lot of pressure when it came to doing well and passing the test. So the last few aspects that we tapped on were the following…

"Even though I feel all this pressure to pass this test, I now choose to let that pressure go, one deep full breath at a time; and feel calm, confident and relaxed about writing this test instead."

"Even though I feel all this pressure to get a good grade on this test, I now choose to let that pressure go, one deep full breath at a time, and feel calm, confident and relaxed about writing this test instead."

"Even though I feel all this pressure from work to pass this test, I now choose to let that pressure go, one deep full breath at a time, and feel calm, confident and relaxed about writing this test instead."

www.TheHiddenSecretsofEFT.com

And then we finally tapped on…

"Even though I feel all this pressure from my parents to pass this test, I now choose to let that pressure go, one deep full breath at a time, and feel calm, confident and relaxed about writing this test instead."

Notice how I walked my client through from the beginning of her day when she needed to travel to the location of the test, all the way through the possibilities of what could go wrong during the test.

By working through the day from start to finish I was able to help her identify and clear all possible aspects!

For other clients who find this type of fear or anxiety seeping into all different areas of their life, I would go back one step further and address *"the earliest memory of this same feeling"*.

This will often take you back to the root cause where you can then tap on all aspects connected to that memory.

www.TheHiddenSecretsofEFT.com

www.TheHiddenSecretsofEFT.com

Ridding the Toxic Relationships in Your Life and Connecting to Love

"Some of the biggest challenges in relationships come from the fact that most people enter a relationship in order to get something. In reality, the only way a relationship will last is if you see your relationship as a place that you go to give, and not a place that you go to take."
~ Anthony Robbins

www.TheHiddenSecretsofEFT.com

www.TheHiddenSecretsofEFT.com

EFT to Enhance Your Relationships

This chapter focuses on relationships we have with others — be it romantic, business, family or friendship.

Generally speaking, we attract certain people into our life for a reason. If undesirable people are turning up in our life that are treating us badly, there are lessons to be learnt around those experiences with those people.

If we don't learn the lesson, we will continue to attract the same pattern of people into different stages of our life.

If we do learn the lesson, these people will no longer be entering our life, and will begin attracting new types of people to learn new lessons.

It's important we focus on the real underlying issues and not play the blame game, pointing the finger at everyone but ourselves. Accepting responsibility for the people in our lives and how they treat us is the key.

Not Being Able to Accept Others

Typically people who accept themselves are more accepting of others, and those who cannot accept themselves often find it easy to find fault with others.

Do you only like certain qualities in people you know and can't bring yourself to accept every bit of them, warts and all?

www.TheHiddenSecretsofEFT.com

Do you wish your brother/friend/husband would look or behave differently? Do you wish your best friend wasn't so beautiful? Do you wish your sister stopped interfering in your life? Or do you wish your husband dressed differently?

Do you withhold love or affection to someone close to you, in an attempt to blackmail them into doing something differently? For example, have you refused to make love with your partner until they have tidied the garage?

The people you attract into your life are largely speaking a reflection of who you are.

So if you find yourself surrounded by many critical people, perhaps you need to resolve the critic within. If on the other hand, you are mostly surrounded by happy, sunny people then you know you're on the right track.

Please tap on the following setup phrases below...

> "Even though I can't accept X exactly the way they are and I wish they would change, I can love and accept myself anyway, fully and completely. I now choose to accept X for who they are, and not how I wish them to be."

> "Even though my husband is perfect in every way apart from the fact he doesn't listen to me, I can love and accept myself anyway, fully and completely. I now choose to turn the tables and ask myself if I am listening and tuning into what he is saying."

> "Even though I'll only be able to accept X when they _____, I can love and accept myself anyway, fully and completely.

I now choose to accept all of X and not just the parts I favor."

"Even though I have great difficulty accepting others as I still can't embrace myself, I can love and accept myself anyway, fully and completely. I now choose to do the best I can in accepting me, knowing the more I accept myself, the more I'm able to accept others."

"Even though X is not good enough and it's so easy for me to find fault with them, ==I can love and accept myself anyway, fully and completely. I now choose to realize that everyone is perfect in their imperfection,== and it would be a boring world if everybody was exactly how I wanted them to be."

"Even though I feel ashamed of X because my friends don't approve of X, I can love and accept myself anyway, fully and completely. I now choose to forgive myself for my negative feelings and accept X for exactly who they are."

"Even though I am so embarrassed when X does _____, and wish they didn't do that, I can love and accept myself anyway, fully and completely. I now choose to be proud of X for being true to themselves and not caring about what others think."

"Even though X doesn't respond to me in the way I'd like them to, I can love and accept myself anyway, fully and completely. I now choose to allow others the freedom to be who they are, without any exceptions."

"Even though I take it personally when X does _____, I can love and accept myself anyway, fully and completely. I now choose to understand that X does _____, not to offend me but because it brings X joy."

www.TheHiddenSecretsofEFT.com

Are You Postponing Happiness?

Too many of us deny happiness, due to not being present in our lives right in this minute. We tell ourselves we are not deserving of happiness until we have reached certain milestones or achieved different things at specific ages.

Too many of us live in the future which always seems to be just out of our reach.

Have you ever told yourself you will only be happy once your children are all in college, once you've bought your own home, or when you meet the "right" person?

It's a shame not to focus on your current relationships, and enjoy where you are right now.

Please tap on the following setup phrases…

> "Even though I won't be happy in my relationship until X proposes to me, I can love and accept myself anyway, fully and completely. I now choose to enjoy this early stage of our relationship whether it progresses further or not."

> "Even though I feel unhappiness as I am stuck caring for my elderly parents, I can love and accept myself anyway, fully and completely. I now choose to be grateful my parents are still alive and find joy in each moment I share with them."

> "Even though X must go to school before I can feel free and happy, I can love and accept myself anyway, fully and completely. I now choose to treasure these years, recognizing every stage of childhood brings its own blessings."

"Even though I have been divorced twice and still haven't found the perfect wo/man to share a romantic relationship with, I can love and accept myself anyway, fully and completely. I now choose to accept myself and be happy, whether I'm in a romantic relationship or not."

"Even though X must happen before I can even think about being happy, I can love and accept myself anyway, fully and completely. I now choose to forgive myself for wasting so much precious time and allow myself to be happy now."

"Even though I have delayed, deterred and prevented happiness in my life for so long, I can love and accept myself anyway, fully and completely. I now choose to allow happiness into my daily life immediately."

I Want to Control Others

Although many of us wouldn't admit that we control others, most of us are guilty of this.

When you suggest to others (without them asking for your advice) what they should think, feel, act and behave, then you are trying to control them.

Perhaps you feel uncomfortable because a certain aspect of someone threatens you in some way. For example, perhaps you don't like the fact your friend is so friendly towards members of the opposite sex and you are jealous of the attention they receive, so you tell your friend they shouldn't act that way.

www.TheHiddenSecretsofEFT.com

Or perhaps you resent the fact your husband seems to have time for everyone but you, which makes you feel inadequate. So you tell him that he doesn't care about or love you. You tell him that if he really loves you, he would act how you want him to act.

These are all examples of wanting to control other people, and if we could stop doing this, most of our relationship problems would be solved.

Please tap on the following setup phrases…

"Even though I have attempted to control those close to me, I can love and accept myself anyway, fully and completely. I now choose to forgive myself and keep my opinions to myself."

"Even though I have told others what to think, what to feel, what to say and how to act, I can love and accept myself anyway, fully and completely. I now choose to allow others the freedom to think, feel, talk and act how they choose, because it is their life, not mine."

"Even though I feel threatened when others are being who they are—because it challenges who I am—I can love and accept myself anyway, fully and completely. I now choose to find out why I feel threatened and dissolve these negative feelings, so I no longer feel threatened."

"Even though I don't like it when others think/talk/look and act differently from me because I feel inadequate, I can love and accept myself anyway, fully and completely. I now

choose to understand that humans are more the same than different, and to look beyond the surface."

I Force My Expectations Onto Others

Sometimes it's hard for us to accept that others must live their own lives and don't need us telling them how to live. It's important we don't place our own expectations on others, as it is their choice to make and not ours.

Demonstrating true unconditional love is just that—not placing conditions or expectations on others.

This section is very important! Please tap on the following setup statements...

> "Even though I place my expectations on others and get angry if they are not fulfilled, I can love and accept myself anyway, fully and completely. I now choose to focus only on having expectations on myself and not on others."

> "Even though I missed out on certain situations, events and experiences and I pushed my children to take advantage of every opportunity I missed out on, I can love and accept myself anyway, fully and completely. I now choose to accept that my children's decisions are their own to make, and I have no right living my dreams through them."

> "Even though I take it personally and get insulted when others don't carry out the expectations I place on them, I can love and accept myself anyway, fully and completely. I now choose

to forgive myself for placing any expectations on anyone, knowing we are all in charge of our own expectations."

"Even though X would do so much better in life if they would just listen to me (because I know best), I can love and accept myself anyway, fully and completely. I now choose to understand that I may not know best, and even if I think I do, it is not my place to tell others how to live their lives—it is up to them, and I now respect that."

"Even though I won't be happy until X does something I want them to do, I can love and accept myself anyway, fully and completely. I now choose to understand that nothing outside of me (including what anybody does or doesn't do) can make me happy. Happiness can only come out of the love I have for myself."

"Even though I want to change how X does something, I can love and accept myself anyway, fully and completely. I now choose to accept others 100% for who and how they are, knowing that I cannot change anyone. Change can only come from within each person."

"Even though I want to make someone fit the ideal I have of them, I can love and accept myself anyway, fully and completely. I now choose to take responsibility for the people I attract into my life. If I don't like the people in my life, it's up to me to make a different choice, instead of forcing someone to be whom they are clearly not."

I Make Others Responsible for My Happiness

It's easy to fall into the trap of making other people in your life responsible for making you happy. Do you feel it is your partner's job to make you happy? Do you burden your children with the heavy weight of your happiness?

It is not respectful or fair to make your husband, wife, child or best friend responsible for your happiness. For all the good and bad in your life, please do not give credit to or blame anyone but yourself.

Your happiness is your responsibility, and yours alone. Please tap on the following setup statements...

"Even though I have put my own happiness in everyone else's hands except my own, I can love and accept myself anyway, fully and completely. I now choose to forgive myself and begin now to accept that happiness is the result of my own love."

"Even though I have told my husband I will only be happy if he gives me another child, I can love and accept myself anyway, fully and completely. I now choose to accept full responsibility for the choices I have made and can still make."

"Even though I will only be happy when all my children finish college and have been accepted into high-paying employment, I can love and accept myself anyway, fully and completely. I now choose to be happy regardless of whether my children go to college or not (or have a well-paying job or not)."

www.TheHiddenSecretsofEFT.com

"Even though I have wrongly assumed happiness can only come from others and has nothing to do with me, I can love and accept myself anyway, fully and completely. I now choose to feel empowered that I control the amount of happiness in my life—whether I allow a little or a lot."

Fear of Rejection If I Reveal My True Self

Are you scared to be who you are? Do you present a false side of yourself to others in the hope that they will like the pretend you? Are you different with different people?

Are you so used to lying to others that you find it hard to know who the real you is?

If you are you trapped in denial and caught up in a web of lies, now is the time to break free.

Please tap on the following setup statements...

"Even though I have spent so long pretending to be someone I'm not (and that I don't even know who I am), I can love and accept myself anyway, fully and completely. I now choose to forgive myself slowly, pull down the facade and reveal the real me."

"Even though I am a people-pleaser and will do anything just so others will like me, I can love and accept myself anyway, fully and completely. I now choose to be true to myself. Other's opinions of me do not matter. All that matters is what I think of myself."

"Even though I am living in a web of lies because social interactions with others are so painful, I can love and accept myself anyway, fully and completely. I now choose to walk away from my lies, with my head held high and live truthfully from now on."

"Even though I am scared to reveal who I really am (because I fear no one will accept me) I can love and accept myself anyway, fully and completely. I now choose to see that the barriers I put up, are only attracting people to the false me and not the real me."

"Even though I am afraid to express what I feel, I can love and accept myself anyway, fully and completely. I now choose to open my heart and to share who I really am, warts and all."

"Even though I fear I am not good enough and will be rejected for who I am, I can love and accept myself anyway, fully and completely. I now choose to seek recognition and validation only from myself and not from other people."

"Even though it doesn't feel safe to be who I am, and it's easier pretending to be someone I'm not, I can love and accept myself anyway, fully and completely. I now choose to see that my life will continue to be a lie until I take the risk of trusting myself to be me."

Practising Forgiveness

Do you still remember the time 20 years ago when X did something to you? Do you still harbor feelings of resentment that the person of your dreams married someone else and not you?

It's important to understand that the action of others is not because of you (or who you are) or anything you may have done, but solely because of them.

Unforgivingness can create stress, anxiety and broken relationships and can create ill-health in the body. Practising forgiveness on a regular basis is healthy for you, and healthy for your relationships.

You will know when EFT has released any negative feelings because you will feel neutral or even compassionate towards those involved. Remember that you are practising forgiveness for you own emotional health and for others.

Please tap on the following setup statements below...

> *"Even though I have held tightly onto painful memories of past hurts as if they happened yesterday, I can love and accept myself anyway, fully and completely. I now choose to forgive myself and anyone else involved, knowing I have the chance now to release any ill feelings."*

> *"Even though I have taken it so personally that X did _____ to me, I can love and accept myself anyway, fully and completely. I now choose to understand that X did what they did because of them and it had nothing to do with me*

at all."

"Even though I can't forget the time when _____ happened, and it's like a black cloud hanging over my life, I can love and accept myself anyway, fully and completely. I now choose to forgive myself and anyone else involved. I trust that everything happens for a reason and to take the lesson from the experience and move on peacefully."

"Even though I feel resentful when I remember _____, I can love and accept myself anyway, fully and completely. I now choose to forgive myself and anyone else involved. I release all ill feelings and replace them with joy and love."

I Can't Help Overreacting

How many times have you kicked yourself for reacting too fast? Have you ever regretted something that you said, or wished you could have behaved differently?

By the time you realized what you had said or done, the damage was already done—too late to undo any actions.

Learning from your mistakes, it's now up to you to practice being more aware and thinking before you speak or act. When someone is trying to say or do something, let it sink into your mind before you go rushing in with your guns blazing.

Listen—don't plan what you are going to say next. Stop and think about what someone is saying. Really concentrate on their words and give them your full attention.

www.TheHiddenSecretsofEFT.com

Once you've taken in, comprehended and really understood what has been said, then take your time in replying. See how you would normally react, and in that moment say something else—something that is supportive and loving, and not critical or judgemental.

The more you actively listen, the more carefully you can respond, instead of mindlessly reacting.

Please tap on the following setup phrases…

"Even though I have blindly reacted to others without stopping to consider the consequences of what I said or did, I can love and accept myself anyway, fully and completely. I now choose to forgive myself and make a conscious effort to be more aware of my interactions with others."

"Even though I have reacted to others blindly, I can love and accept myself anyway, fully and completely. I now choose to respond with love."

"Even though I have hurt others in the past for speaking or acting without thinking, I can love and accept myself anyway, fully and completely. I now choose to forgive myself and anyone else involved, and practice being more aware."

"Even though I feel sad because my life would have turned out differently had I responded differently in various situations, I can love and accept myself anyway, fully and completely. I now choose to turn my attention to the present moment, knowing I can influence my future by what I think, say and do today."

"Even though I've probably never listened properly to others before, I can love and accept myself anyway, fully and completely. I now choose to actively listen today and every day, knowing the more I practice, the better I will become. It is never too late to initiate the gift of listening."

The Freedom to Make New Choices

During days where you feel stuck or don't know which way to turn in your relationships with others, it's comforting to know you can always do something about it.

For simplicity, there are only two real choices when you are in a situation you don't like that involves others.

You can either accept the situation as it is or you can leave it. Do not stick around hoping to change that person, their opinions or their actions, as it'll be a waste of time.

For example, if your close friend who you have known for years and years has betrayed you in some way, ask yourself how you feel?

If you feel you can move on from the betrayal and that your friendship still has a lot of love in it, then forgive your friend and accept they made a mistake. Do not punish them or make them feel any worse than they do by bringing the betrayal up time and time again.

If on the other hand you simply cannot accept what they've done, it is therefore time to move on and not involve that

www.TheHiddenSecretsofEFT.com

friend in your life anymore. Explain your feelings to them, wish them happiness, and then move on quietly without them.

Let's say, one of your relationships is simply growing apart, rather than some dramatic incident occurring (such as, a partner cheating on you), how would this make you feel?

If you feel sad, see if you can find new ways to inject renewed intimacy into your relationship. If on the other hand you feel relieved when you consider that person not being in your life, then follow your heart and distance yourself from that relationship.

Remember that you always have a choice, especially in situations where you don't feel like there is one.

Please tap on the following setup phrases…

"Even though I feel I am stuck in a dead-end friendship with X, I can love and accept myself anyway, fully and completely. I now choose to realize I have the freedom to choose whether to accept things as they are or move on."

"Even though I don't know what to do about _____ situation with my child, I can love and accept myself anyway, fully and completely. I now choose to forgive and forget, starting a new day."

"Even though I am completely undecided about whether to accept things as they are or move away from my relationship with X, I can love and accept myself anyway, fully and completely. I now choose to be open to the right choice."

"Even though I cannot forget what X has done and it's straining our relationship, I can love and accept myself anyway, fully and completely. I now choose to dissolve any negativity until I feel neutral about the situation."

"Even though it doesn't feel like I have a choice, I can love and accept myself anyway, fully and completely. I now choose to trust that no matter what I do, I'll always have a choice and it is mine alone to make."

Expressing and Receiving Love

There are many books out there dedicated to making sense of the different ways we give and receive love. Are you aware of your love language?

Often how we express our love for others is the same as how we want to feel loved.

For example, you may show your love for your family by cooking meals, cleaning the house and mending clothes. In return you may feel loved when your children do the washing up or your husband mows the lawn.

Or perhaps you like to show your affection for those in your life by giving presents. In return you may also enjoy receiving gifts and feel unloved if those close to you don't express their love for you in this way.

It is a case of finding out how you demonstrate your love for others and being honest about what makes you feel loved.

www.TheHiddenSecretsofEFT.com

You may become dissatisfied if those close to you don't love you in the same way you would like to feel loved.

So you ask X to do the things that make you feel loved; however, that can become a problem, as X may not express love in that way— it may be unnatural for them to do that. Person X may become resentful for being told how to act.

You may have to ask yourself if there are any areas you can be flexible in? If not, do you have the right to ask someone to be something they're not? Would you like it if someone asked this of you? The answer is probably not!

It's easier to be with those who already show, demonstrate and express love the way you like, than to force someone to act in a way that suits you.

This section mostly applies to your romantic relationships, as this person plays a vital role in your life.

So what do you do when you and your partner communicate in a different love language? You can either accept them and the way they express love, or you can leave this relationship and choose someone else who you feel more compatible with.

Please tap on the following setup phrases...

> *"Even though my partner and I have different ways of expressing love, I can love and accept myself anyway, fully and completely. I now choose to look at my options and make a choice that feels right for me, knowing that I deserve to feel loved."*

"Even though I can't accept the way my partner expresses their love to me, and I don't want to leave our relationship, I can love and accept myself anyway, fully and completely. I now choose to listen to my heart, for the solution lies inside of me."

"Even though I don't feel loved by my partner and I think it is their entire fault, I can love and accept myself anyway, fully and completely. I now choose to realize there are two people in a relationship, and if I'm not feeling loved then probably neither is my partner."

"Even though I'll never find someone who will love me the way I like to feel loved, I can love and accept myself anyway, fully and completely. I now choose to concentrate on loving myself, trusting the right person will come along at the perfect time."

Case Study

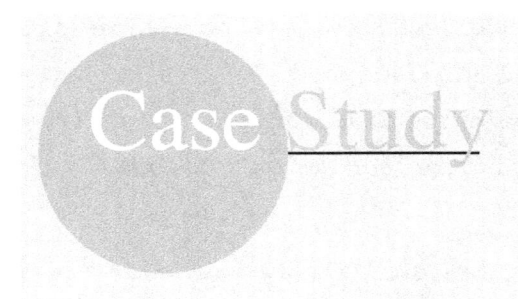

Relationship problems often involve many different aspects and accompanying emotions. Even though everyone has their own personal relationship problems to work through, I often see similar emotions surfacing.

Below is a great example of how rapidly emotions shift and change. It's also a great example of how to use EFT methodically and practically, to quickly get to the heart of the problem.

A client came to me obviously angry, so there was no need to do a generic round of tapping.

So we started at...

"Even though I feel infuriated as I can't be who I am when I'm with my husband, I now choose to sense my feelings — perhaps for the first time in a long time."

We then tapped on...

"Even though I feel silenced in the presence of my husband and I can't express myself, I now choose to let my feelings surface."

She then stated she didn't feel a connection with her husband, so we tapped on…

"Even though I don't feel there is any intimacy or loving connection between us, I choose now to see my situation honestly."

And then her thoughts shifted to…

"Even though I know I deserve to be in a relationship where I can be who I am and be loved and accepted for this, I now choose to believe I am deserving of this."

My client's thoughts then changed to…

"Even though I feel trapped and confused because I'm in a relationship where I cannot accept how things are, and I cannot leave, I now choose to have clarity."

At this point, I asked my client why she couldn't leave her husband—what was stopping her? So we tapped on her fear…

"Even though I am scared to leave my safe, comfortable relationship; but know deep down there is no way I can put up with my feelings of being trapped, I now choose to release this fear."

After that, I asked her how she felt? We then tapped on…

"Even though I feel overwhelmed by the enormity of the consequences if I were to leave this relationship, I choose now to face these consequences with love and grace."

Gently, I asked my client what she felt were the huge consequences she would have to face if she were to leave her husband? She blurted out four very different reasons, which we tapped on separately...

"Even though I don't want to end this relationship because I can't face the upheaval and feel overwhelmed at the thought, I choose now to feel peaceful."

After tapping on this thought, my client told me that she had ended relationships in the past, and whilst it was disruptive, she came out the other end stronger and happier.

So we moved onto the next consequence...

"Even though I don't want to end this relationship because I'm scared of what my family and society will think about me, I can love and accept myself anyway, fully and completely."

And...

"Even though I think it's a failure if I were to be a single mother (and I don't like this stigma), I can love and accept myself anyway, fully and completely."

After tapping on those two thoughts regarding what others may have thought about her, my client told me that everyone could think what they liked and she felt peaceful about it.

Next, we tapped on another consequence of leaving her marriage...

"Even though I don't want to end the relationship because then I will have to be financially responsible for myself and my 18 month old baby, I now choose to feel hopeful."

Her beliefs of feeling daunted and weighted down by financial responsibility changed, as she told me she had always wanted to be 100% independent and this would be her chance.

We then tapped on her final objection regarding leaving her husband…

"Even though I don't want to end this relationship because I want a way out that is easy and with minimal disruption (one that I don't think is possible), I now choose to face the reality."

Her feelings of being stuck shifted, to feeling confident and having the strength to leave her husband. By the end of the session, my client told me that it felt right to leave her husband. She said that it was better to be with someone who accepted her for who she was, rather than forcing her husband to be how she wanted him to be.

www.TheHiddenSecretsofEFT.com

Release Your Emotions, Release Your Fat

"The big secret in life is that there is no big secret.
Whatever your goal, you can get there
if you're willing to work."
~ Oprah Winfrey

www.TheHiddenSecretsofEFT.com

Weight Loss

Carrying excess weight can result in serious health problems, including the cause of many illnesses.

Diabetes, certain cancers, and spinal and heart problems, have all been blamed on the increase of people who consume an unhealthy diet.

The cost to our health services is phenomenal, and most governments in the Western World have implemented healthier eating programs in communities and schools.

Most people would agree, that being overweight is an emotional problem.

Too many diet companies claim their latest and greatest diet program is the one that will guarantee weight loss.

Unfortunately, the real issue that is causing the weight gain is not being addressed, so any weight that is lost is usually only temporary.

When you use EFT to address and heal the real reasons why you have excess weight, you will experience permanent results.

If you have been on the dieting treadmill, the following routine will be all too familiar… You eat, you diet, you fail with your new diet, you then feel bad and comfort yourself with more food, and then begin a new diet.

This cycle of behavior is destructive for your self-esteem and dangerous for your health.

Being Overweight is Part of My Identity

If you have always been overweight, it is likely that being "fat" is part of who you think you are. It is part of how you identify yourself.

Probably for as long as you can remember you have been the "fat child", and perhaps were even chubby as a baby.

You may feel powerless to change how you are because you believe you have "fat genes".

You may accept your family history and take comfort in the fact that your mother and father are big too. You may even use this as an excuse to hide and avoid trying to lose weight, even though you know the eating patterns you've copied from your parents are not healthy.

Please tap on the following setup phrases…

> *"Even though for as long as I can remember I've been fat and it's part of who I am (and it's all I know), I can love and accept myself anyway, fully and completely. I now choose to be open to a new identity where I am healthier and slimmer."*

> *"Even though I can't help how I am because I have fat genes and it's not my fault, I can love and accept myself anyway, fully and completely. I now choose to forgive my parents for giving me a predisposition to being overweight, take responsibility for being healthier, and not use my parents as an excuse."*

"Even though there is no hope for me to ever be slim, and I just have to accept that I'll always be fat, I can love and accept myself anyway, fully and completely. I now choose to take a more empowering approach to my health and not give up so easily."

"Even though all my family are large, and if I were to lose weight they wouldn't love me anymore, I can love and accept myself anyway, fully and completely. I now choose to accept that I may encounter criticism for not staying the same as them, but I choose to put my health and well-being ahead of their opinions."

"Even though I just can't imagine myself being any different, as being fat is all I've ever known, I can love and accept myself anyway, fully and completely. I now choose to accept that it's OK to feel uncomfortable, knowing that my discomfort will ease the more I get used to the idea of a healthier me."

Lack of Self-Esteem

Many root reasons for being overweight stem from a lack of self-esteem—not feeling good enough or not feeling you are deserving of something. Not loving and accepting yourself for who you are all contribute to low self-esteem.

Perhaps someone said something to you and you believed what they said about you to be true. Perhaps you grew up in a home where you felt that nothing you did was ever good enough. Or perhaps you have always found fault with yourself from a young age.

www.TheHiddenSecretsofEFT.com

Cast your mind back to the first time you felt unworthy, unloved or not good enough. What or who led you to believe these thoughts? Tap on this scenario, forgiving anyone involved and clearing all negative emotions.

Please use the following setup statements as examples for your own…

"Even though my dad told me I was useless and would never amount to anything, I can love and accept myself anyway, fully and completely. I now choose to forgive him for saying that and myself for believing him. I now realize his words were not true."

"Even though everything I did when I was young seemed to be wrong, I can love and accept myself anyway, fully and completely. I now choose to forgive my parents, and understand they had problems that were nothing to do with me."

"Even though I have always been critical and unloving towards myself, I can love and accept myself anyway, fully and completely. I now choose to see that I am perfect within my imperfections."

"Even though I feel unworthy/ashamed/undeserving of being loved by myself, I can love and accept myself anyway, fully and completely. I now choose to realize it is never too late to start loving, and looking after myself today."

"Even though I hate myself because _____ and I turned to food for comfort, I can love and accept myself anyway, fully and completely. I now choose to forgive myself and anyone else involved."

"Even though food has always been there for me when _____ wasn't, I can love and accept myself anyway, fully and completely. I now choose to recognize that eating will not make me feel emotionally full, only self-love will."

Being Overweight to Protect Yourself

Perhaps part of the reason you are overweight is to protect yourself from certain people or situations you are afraid of.

Were you ever teased as a child or called names? Do you ever wish you were invisible? Do you shy away from relationships with the opposite sex?

If so, perhaps unconsciously you have gained weight to put up a wall of protection that keeps others away from you—and perhaps this suits you. Or perhaps being big is the way you punish others.

There are many possibilities. Even if they don't seem to make sense, your reasons are real for you. Let's explore what some of them may be. Tap on the following setup phrases...

"Even though I am so shy and don't want others to get to know me (so I have kept people away by being big), I can love and accept myself anyway, fully and completely. I now choose to realize that the world is missing out by not knowing me. It is safe for me to be who I am."

"Even though the kids at school called me names and I wanted to show them their words didn't affect me (so I ate and ate), I can love and accept myself anyway, fully and completely. I now choose to forgive those kids and myself for believing them. I know that my past doesn't dictate my future."

"Even though I am afraid of X, so I've gained weight to prevent me from facing X, I can love and accept myself anyway, fully and completely. I now choose to explore why I feel so afraid and dissolve my fears one by one."

"Even though I am wary of being in a romantic relationship with the opposite sex, I can love and accept myself anyway, fully and completely. I now choose to trust others, knowing I am deserving of giving and receiving love."

"Even though I am ashamed of who I am, and have literally put up a wall of protection around me in terms of extra weight, I can love and accept myself anyway, fully and completely. I now choose to love and accept myself more each day."

"Even though I enjoy the many advantages of being overweight, I can love and accept myself anyway, fully and completely. I now choose to understand the benefits of being healthier, far outweigh any benefits of being big."

I Turned to Food to Help Me Through a Difficult Time

We all go through periods in our lives that are stressful, difficult and sad. Often when we feel overwhelmed we turn to food for a quick fix.

Enjoying the quick lift we feel, we then return to eating over and over. Soon we are in a habit of eating for comfort rather than fueling our bodies.

There may be specific foods we turn to or we may consume, just to feel full. There may be times when it is difficult to feel our emotions and we over-eat until we are stuffed, just so we can feel *something*.

Have a think about any events that happened in your life that led you to comfort eat. What emotions did you feel at the time? It could be that now, whenever you feel that particular emotion, it triggers you to comfort-eat.

Please use the following setup statements below as examples for your own situation…

> *"Even though when I got divorced, I turned to sugary food to try to ease the bitterness inside me, I can love and accept myself anyway, fully and completely. I now choose to forgive my partner, dissolving any bitterness I feel."*

> *"Even though an increase in my income has seen me buying more luxurious and unhealthy foods, I can love and accept myself anyway, fully and completely. I now choose to spend my money more wisely, on healthier alternatives that will nourish my body and mind."*

> *"Even though my eating became erratic when X died (sometimes I ate nothing and other times I binged), I can love and accept myself anyway, fully and completely. I now choose to listen to my body and eat only when I am hungry."*

www.TheHiddenSecretsofEFT.com

"Even though my job position has changed, and I have to entertain clients over big lunches and dinners (where I always indulge as work pays), I can love and accept myself anyway, fully and completely. I now choose to stop using this as an excuse, as there are plenty of healthy items on the menu I can order."

"Even though I turn to chocolate whenever I am sad, upset or angry, I can love and accept myself anyway, fully and completely. I now choose to substitute my behavior by eating something healthy."

Uncontrollable Food Cravings

Do you crave certain foods at certain times in the day? Can you not face the start of each day without strong coffee and sugar to start the day? In the middle of the afternoon do you find yourself reaching for a fatty snack to rectify an energy slump?

Is it automatic for you to watch TV whilst munching unhealthy snacks? Can you only talk on the telephone when you've got a hot sweet drink in front of you?

If any of those sound familiar to you, please tap on the following setup statements…

"Even though I cannot get up in the morning without caffeine and sugar, I can love and accept myself anyway, fully and completely. I now choose to fill my body with life-giving and not life-depleting foods."

"Even though I skip breakfast, but by morning tea I am famished and reach for a slice of cake for an instant lift, I can love and accept myself anyway, fully and completely. I now choose to eat a healthy breakfast, and if I am still hungry choose a healthy snack."

"Even though I have a huge slump in energy in the middle of the afternoon and instantly reach for chocolate, I can love and accept myself anyway, fully and completely. I now choose to change this unhealthy habit and choose something healthy."

"Even though I cannot watch TV without devouring a huge packet of chips, I can love and accept myself anyway, fully and completely. I now choose to listen to my body, and only eat when I am truly hungry and not just out of habit."

"Even though when I talk on the phone I like to curl up with coffee and sugar, I can love and accept myself anyway, fully and completely. I now choose to drink water if I am thirsty."

"Even though when I carry out certain tasks I like to have my favorite foods or drinks with me, I can love and accept myself anyway, fully and completely. I now choose to forgive myself and decide to break my habits today."

"Even though I crave and need to eat chocolate every day, I can love and accept myself anyway, fully and completely. I now choose to be open to finding out the root of this emotional eating."

"Even though I crave X food and I don't think I can live without it, I can love and accept myself anyway, fully and completely. I now choose to release any emotional connection I've associated with the food I crave."

I Can't Stop Eating

Would you say you are addicted to eating? Do you only feel happy when you are about to eat, you are eating or you've just finished eating?

Are you unable to stop yourself eating, as if when you are in the presence of food you cannot control yourself?

Do you eat like a mad wo/man because you are so ashamed of your eating? Do you consume food so quickly so you can trick yourself into believing your frenzied eating episode never happened?

Do you make excuses and keep eating, just because you have started eating? For example, you might eat a piece of cake, and then think you've broken the diet you're on, so you have another piece and then another…

If you can relate to any of these, please tap on the following setup phrases…

> "Even though I am addicted to eating everything and anything, and I feel so helpless, I can love and accept myself anyway, fully and completely. I now choose to forgive myself and be open to the root cause of my addiction, so I can resolve each issue layer by layer."
>
> "Even though the only time I feel happy is when food is near me, I can love and accept myself anyway, fully and completely. I

now choose to build my happiness from within, knowing true happiness cannot be sought from external things."

"Even though when I overeat I wolf down everything in sight as quickly as I can (because I am so ashamed of what I am doing), I can love and accept myself anyway, fully and completely. I now choose to taste, enjoy and savor the food I eat from now on."

"Even though I feel out of control and hate myself for eating so much, I can love and accept myself anyway, fully and completely. I now choose to forgive myself and trust that EFT will help me heal my negative feelings."

"Even though when I've started to eat something I feel I have to eat all of it, right then and there, I can love and accept myself anyway, fully and completely. I now choose to listen to my body and eat as much as my body needs."

Binge Eating

Do you starve yourself for long periods when you skip meals and then indulge in an enormous amount of food later to make up for it?

Do you stick to your diet and then on day 3 break it, letting all intentions fly out the window as you eat and eat and eat?

Do you eat at night in secret, so no-one discovers what you are up to? Do you wake in the night at a certain time—as if by clock-work—unable to return to sleep until you've raided the pantry?

If so, please use any of the following examples as setup phrases to tap on…

"Even though I restrict my food intake considerably only to lose control later, I can love and accept myself anyway, fully and completely. I now choose to forgive myself and release my "all or nothing" attitude, and indulge a little in the foods I like without going overboard."

"Even though I have such high aspirations which I can't follow through on, I can love and accept myself anyway, fully and completely. I now choose to lower my goals so they are realistic and achievable. I can always raise them as I move forward."

"Even though I hate it when I gorge on food, I can love and accept myself anyway, fully and completely. I now choose to forgive myself and uncover the root reason I am emotionally hungry."

"Even though I don't know why I binge eat, I can love and accept myself anyway, fully and completely. I now choose to reflect on my past and see if there was a time in my life when this unhealthy eating started."

"Even though I'm ashamed how much I eat (so I eat when no one else is home), I can love and accept myself anyway, fully and completely. I now choose to forgive myself for my behavior and be open to stopping it now."

"Even though I eat in my sleep, has been a habit for years and is part of my life I can love and accept myself anyway, fully and completely. I now choose to be open to resolving and ceasing my night eating once and for all."

Emotional Eating

Most eating problems are linked to our emotions. When you can address the root emotional problem that underlies your unhealthy eating, your problems with food will cease too.

Do you use food as a reward? Have you ever felt deprived in the past and you eat and eat to feel emotionally full? Do you feel empty, lonely or unloved? Do you use food to fill that hole?

There are so many emotional causes to eating, so it's important you uncover your own as they will be personal to you.

Tap on the following setup phrases and see what comes up. Continue to follow through until you get to the root cause.

> "Even though no one loves me, and food is always there for me, I can love and accept myself anyway, fully and completely. I now choose to understand that love comes from within and not from someone else loving me."
>
> "Even though I use food to reward myself, and eat and drink in excess when I celebrate something, I can love and accept myself anyway, fully and completely. I now choose a different form of reward to treat myself, instead of using food."
>
> "Even though I eat compulsively whenever I feel sad/happy/angry/frustrated, I can love and accept myself anyway, fully

and completely. I now choose to eat just to fuel my body, and not link certain emotions to eating certain foods."

"Even though I felt so deprived when _____ happened, and I now eat to make up for that situation, I can love and accept myself anyway, fully and completely. I now choose to forgive myself and anyone else involved, dissolving all feelings of deprivation now."

"Even though I don't feel good enough and I eat to feel better, I can love and accept myself anyway, fully and completely. I now choose to nurture myself with self-love, and not turn to food to fill me up emotionally."

www.TheHiddenSecretsofEFT.com

Case Study

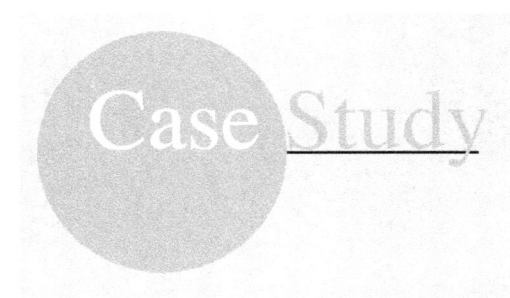

Below is a great example with one particular client, who worked through the many layers of specific food issues that were preventing her from losing weight.

We started tapping with...

"Even though my weight has reached a plateau and I can't seem to get past it, I love and accept myself anyway and choose now to feel comfortable at my goal weight."

I asked my client to think about what it would feel like to actually be at her goal weight, and she stated that it didn't feel comfortable for a few different reasons.

Once we identified them, we started tapping on the following...

"Even though I have a block to weighing less than 150 pounds, I love and accept myself anyway and choose to feel comfortable at my goal weight instead."

"Even though I don't feel comfortable weighing less than 150 pounds because men might find me attractive, I love and accept myself anyway, and choose to feel comfortable and safe at my goal weight instead."

And then we tapped on...

"Even though I don't know who I'd really be if I were to weigh less than 150 pounds, I love and accept myself anyway, and choose to feel comfortable at my goal weight instead."

"Even though I sabotage myself whenever I weigh less than 150 pounds, I love and accept myself anyway and choose to feel comfortable at my goal weight."

As she started to feel more safe and comfortable with the idea of weighing her goal weight, we then moved on to understanding her relationship with food and her reasons for overeating.

I asked her about the times when she normally over ate, what emotions she thought would come up if she stopped that habit? We then tapped on the statements below...

"Even though I overeat to avoid my feelings, I love and forgive myself fully and completely. I now choose to change my behavior and eat only what my body needs."

"Even though I overeat when I'm lonely, I love and forgive myself fully and completely. I now choose to begin to feel my emotions instead."

"Even though I overeat when I'm sad, I love and forgive myself fully and completely. I now choose to begin to feel my emotions instead."

> "Even though I overeat when I'm frustrated, I love and forgive myself fully and completely. I now choose to begin to feel my emotions and also release them."

Once we had cleared all the emotions she was avoiding to feel with food, I then asked my client again to picture herself at her goal weight and notice any feelings that were coming up.

She was able to identify the fact, that deep down, she did not feel worthy or deserving of being at her goal weight.

So we tapped on…

> "Even though I overeat because I think I'm worthless, I love and accept myself anyway and now choose to begin feeling worthy of my goal weight instead."

> "Even though I don't deserve to be happy with my body because I never have been, I love and accept myself anyway. I now choose to begin feeling that I deserve to be happy instead."

And then we tapped on…

> "Even though I believe I don't deserve to be thin, I choose now to feel deserving instead, trusting and knowing that it's possible for me."

Finally, we decided to focus the last few rounds on forgiving herself for being this way and getting to this point, so that she could let go of the anger towards herself.

We tapped on…

"Even though I'm angry at myself for becoming this way, I now choose to let that go and forgive myself for the mistakes I've made, knowing that I can change from this point forward."

And then we finally tapped on…

"Even though I'm angry that I let myself overeat, I now choose to forgive myself completely, knowing that I can change from this point forward and feel good at my goal weight."

This is a detailed example of how complex weight issues can be. Please keep in mind that your own reasons might be very different, but have just as many aspects/layers. It's important to keep tapping and peeling back the layers to find out the root of the issue.

Busting the Top 8 Smoking Myths — So You Can Stop Smoking Permanently

"One thousand Americans stop smoking every day — by dying."
~ Author Unknown

www.TheHiddenSecretsofEFT.com

Using EFT to Stop Smoking

We all know that smoking is addictive. It is also extremely harmful to your health and the health of others around you.

On average, about 1000 people give up every day. Twice this number attempt to give up, but are unsuccessful. If you are a smoker and want to stop smoking, EFT can help you kick your habit painlessly and permanently.

EFT breaks your association of wanting to smoke with your key emotional triggers. This is something that willpower alone cannot do.

Tap on the following setup phrases to start on your non-smoking journey...

"Even though I don't know what emotional driver led me to smoke in the first place, I deeply and completely love and accept myself. I choose to trust in the process of EFT, and allow whatever feelings I have to surface so I can address them."

"Even though I tried to stop smoking in the past and I failed, (and I'm sure I'll fail again), I deeply and completely love and accept myself. I choose to accept that my past doesn't define me and to concentrate only on the present moment."

"Even though I am too addicted to smoking to stop, and I doubt that EFT will work for me, I deeply and completely love and accept myself. I choose to be open to the possibility that EFT may work, even if I think it's new-age nonsense."

www.TheHiddenSecretsofEFT.com

"Even though I don't know if I want to stop smoking or not, I deeply and completely love and accept myself. I choose to stop only when I truly feel ready. I choose to accept my decision to stop smoking whether it's today, tomorrow or in 10 years."

"Even though I know smoking is bad for my health and could kill me, I deeply and completely love and accept myself. I choose to be open-minded about the many emotional triggers of smoking and will eradicate them, one by one."

"Even though I feel like a failure for continuing to smoke, I deeply and completely love and accept myself. I choose to know that once I'm free of my emotional triggers, so too will my desire to smoke."

Willpower and Smoking

There is no point using willpower alone to give up smoking. This is because you will still have the urge, cravings and desire to smoke no matter how hard you try.

Using willpower alone will only put you through unnecessary misery for months or years. It's not nice forcing yourself to give up, when deep down you still want to smoke.

If you used to smoke and gave up through willpower alone, you will benefit from reading this chapter. You will be able to totally free any remaining deep rooted desire to smoke.

Tap on the following setup phrases to be free from any current beliefs you may have about willpower...

"Even though I have felt to be a complete and utter failure in the past because I wasn't strong enough to stop smoking, I deeply and completely love and accept myself. I choose to forgive myself for wrongly believing that willpower alone is all I needed to stop smoking."

"Even though I have felt like I was living a lie, because I told everyone I didn't have cigarette cravings anymore when I actually did, I deeply and completely love and accept myself. I choose to understand that as long as the desire to smoke is still there, then I haven't emotionally stopped smoking."

"Even though society tells me that I am weak because I have no willpower, I deeply and completely love and accept myself. I choose to accept that I can easily stop smoking without the need for willpower, as soon as I disengage myself from my emotional triggers."

"Even though I believe you have to be emotionally strong-willed to give up smoking and I'm weak, I deeply and completely love and accept myself. I choose to understand that I don't need to be strong-willed at all to stop smoking—I just have to be willing."

"Even though I still believe willpower is a vital part of stopping smoking, I deeply and completely love and accept myself. I choose to be open to the possibility that willpower is not needed at all to give up smoking."

Smoking Language

The words you use have a powerful emotional affect on your actions. Be more aware of the language you use and substitute "weak" words for more empowering words.

Telling others and telling yourself that you want to "quit" smoking can have negative emotions associated with it. The word "quit" has implications of loss and doing something you may not want to do.

Perhaps you tell yourself and others that you are "giving up" smoking. "Giving up" sounds like you are relinquishing something you really don't want to stop doing. "Giving up" sounds weak, as if you are doomed to fail right from the beginning.

Instead of "quitting" or "giving up" smoking, tell yourself and others that you want to stop smoking.

This is a much stronger and more active word. The word "stop" implies strength, finality and freedom from doing something previously—in this case smoking.

"Even though the words I used when I told others I wanted to stop smoking, may have kept me smoking, I deeply and completely love and accept myself. I choose to consciously speak more empowering words about stopping smoking.

Smoking Excuses

If you smoke, you may tell yourself there are many reasons why you do. Some may be more obvious to you, whilst others may be more hidden or subconscious.

Let's tap on some general smoking excuses...

> *"Even though I have told myself every conceivable reason why I smoke, I deeply and completely love and accept myself. I choose to let go of all my excuses easily and permanently."*

> *"Even though I feel afraid to let go of my excuses because I feel safe and familiar with them, I deeply and completely love and accept myself. I choose to trust in the EFT process of gently letting them go, one by one"*

> *"Even though I really believe the reasons why I smoke, and I don't want to let them go (because I don't like to be wrong), I deeply and completely love and accept myself. I choose to believe that it is OK to be wrong sometimes, and that I'm not a bad person because of it."*

Perhaps you smoke because it is part of who you are. Perhaps you smoke because you think it is sociable, or that it helps you to relax, concentrate or cope with stress.

Or perhaps you smoke because you believe it gives you pleasure, keeps you thin, or you simply cannot stop because your cravings are too strong.

We will address all of the above excuses one by one...

www.TheHiddenSecretsofEFT.com

Myth #1 Smoking is My Identity

If you smoke, you know the health risks. You know there's a pile of medical evidence that cigarettes can kill you—but you still choose to smoke.

Your identity as a smoker may be so deeply ingrained that you may feel it is too emotionally painful to break free from. Smoking may define who you are as a person. And the thought of not knowing who you are if you stopped smoking, is a very real concern.

Tap on the following setup phrases to break away from your identity as a smoker...

"Even though I won't know who I am if I stop smoking, I deeply and completely love and accept myself. I choose to form a new identity that doesn't revolve around smoking."

"Even though I'm scared to death of having a new identity as a non-smoker, I deeply and completely love and accept myself. I choose to accept that I won't be a brand new person overnight, and that the process will be gradual and comfortable."

"Even though I feel left out at the thought of giving up smoking—as a big part of my identity is tied up in smoking, I deeply and completely love and accept myself. I choose to gracefully let go of that part of me, that I no longer want anything to do with."

"Even though I will be shunned, ridiculed and excluded from co-smokers (and I desperately want their approval), I deeply

and completely love and accept myself. I choose to accept my new identity of being a non-smoker. If those who smoke cannot support my new decision, then they're not good friends anyway."

"Even though a part of me doesn't want to give up who I am, and I am sad to lose this part of me, I deeply and completely love and accept myself. I choose to move forward slowly, reinventing myself each day."

"Even though I love being different, a bit wild and smoking allowed me to rebel against society, I deeply and completely love and accept myself. I choose to understand I can still stand out from the crowd without having to smoke."

Myth #2 Smoking is Sociable

In the past, people smoked as it was socially acceptable; however, it's unacceptable in our society today. Many restaurants, work-places and public spaces are now smoke-free. There are so many social places where smoking is banned.

Smoking is not sociable! In fact, it is probably one of the most unsociable and anti-social activities you can undertake.

Why would you want the stench of cigarette smoke in your hair, clothes and in your home? Why would you want yellowing teeth, smoker's breath and that hacking, morning cough?

The truth is, smoking is like any other addiction. It is a crutch to help you during times of stress or to prop up insecurities.

Use these setup phrases to tap away the belief that smoking is sociable...

> "Even though I feel insecure in social situations and I believe smoking gives me more confidence, I deeply and completely love and accept myself. I choose to accept that self confidence comes from within and not from a smoking habit."

> "Even though I feel comfortable joining a group of smokers where I am instantly accepted, I deeply and completely love and accept myself. I choose to socialize with others who accept me for who I am, and not whether I smoke or not."

> "Even though there is an unspoken bond between those who smoke—and I like that instant and unspoken connection—I deeply and completely love and accept myself. I choose to understand the superficiality of the bond, and know that it is based on insecurity and not anything deeper."

> "Even though I desperately need smoking as my social crutch and I don't know how I'd cope without my cigarettes, I deeply and completely love and accept myself. I choose to accept I may feel uncomfortable for a short time, while I adjust and gain real self-assurance without my cigarettes."

> "Even though I fear I won't be accepted in social situations by other smokers and be an outcast, I deeply and completely love and accept myself. I choose to understand their reaction, as they may feel threatened by my new non-smoking status."

Myth #3 Smoking Helps Me Relax

The long held belief that smoking is a relaxing pastime is not, and cannot be true.

The myth that smoking helps you relax, is probably the most common held belief that you may have about your habit.

Nicotine is a powerful stimulant. On entering the bloodstream, its effect is almost immediate.

One of the side effects noticed within 30-90 minutes of smoking, is a pharmacologically induced sense of fear.

This artificial fear can only be reduced by smoking another cigarette. It is the feeling of anxiety caused by the nicotine that is being reduced, not any *real* anxiety.

Unfortunately, your subconscious mind believes the stress is caused by real anxiety, and not caused by nicotine.

Now you know the truth—smoking causes anxiety.

Tap on the following setup phrases to remove your belief that smoking helps you relax...

> *"Even though I believe smoking relaxes me, I deeply and completely love and accept myself. I choose to see the truth— that smoking causes anxiety and tension inside my body."*
>
> *"Even though I desperately need a cigarette to relax—and can't relax until one is in my hand, I deeply and completely love and accept myself. I choose to understand that my anxiety will only continue as long as I continue to smoke."*

"Even though my subconscious mind is unable to make the connection between smoking and its delayed effects of stress, I deeply and completely love and accept myself. I choose to be open to accepting the truth."

"Even though I don't want to accept the real truth about smoking causing anxiety, I deeply and completely love and accept myself. I choose to be open-minded enough to believe the reality."

"Even though I don't know how I will relax or what I can do instead of smoking to relax, I deeply and completely love and accept myself. I choose to accept there are other ways I can relax, and smoking is not the only solution."

Myth #4 Smoking Helps Me Concentrate

Unfortunately, smoking doesn't help with concentration or focus. In fact, smoking impairs your concentration.

Your oxygen flow slows down in your body, and your oxygen level is reduced. This results in reduced levels of nutrients and oxygen reaching your brain. Waste products are not only increased, but harder to remove.

Smoking is a habit and an addiction. Breaking your habit and addiction via EFT, will enable you to concentrate just as successfully without smoking.

Beliefs are powerful—even when they are false. When you associate your ability to concentrate with smoking, it is just a misguided belief that has taken over you.

To help your subconscious mind remove the association of

concentration with smoking, please tap on the following...

"Even though it is a great shock and surprise to discover that smoking doesn't help me concentrate, I deeply and completely love and accept myself. I choose to absorb this new truth with an open mind."

"Even though I still firmly believe smoking helps me concentrate—and this belief is very true for me, I deeply and completely love and accept myself. I choose to accept that sometimes beliefs can be wrong, perhaps even this one."

"Even though I must smoke to help me concentrate, I deeply and completely love and accept myself. I choose to recognize the truth that smoking hinders my concentration."

"Even though my subconscious mind still associates the need to smoke with the need to concentrate, I deeply and completely love and accept myself. I choose to forgive myself for falsely associating these things."

"Even though I can't think of other ways to help me concentrate aside from smoking, I deeply and completely love and accept myself. I choose to believe I won't need another crutch to help me focus and concentrate."

"Even though I am angry at myself for believing that smoking helps me concentrate, when it doesn't, I deeply and completely love and accept myself. I choose to be grateful I now know the truth, and not waste time dwelling on the past."

Myth #5 Smoking Helps Me Deal With Stress

This is another common misconception that smoking helps you deal better with stressful situations.

Although smoking may appear to give you temporary relief when you smoke the next cigarette, it is an illusion that smoking helps you overcome stress.

Smoking depletes vitamin C from your body. And you need vitamin C to produce stress response hormones. If you don't have the right amount of vitamin C, you will feel even more stressed.

You are likely to have certain triggers in times of stress that encourage you to reach for your cigarettes.

It is vital you tap on these triggers to remove the association of smoking in stressful situations for you.

Here are some suggestions for your setup phrases...

> *"Even though I still believe that smoking does help me deal with stress, I deeply and completely love and accept myself. I choose to accept the truth... the more I smoke the more I am starving my body of vitamin C and the more stressed I will feel."*

> *"Even though I feel at a loss without my cigarettes to help support me in stressful situations, I deeply and completely love and accept myself. I choose to have the courage to face short-term discomfort whilst my body adjusts to me not smoking anymore."*

"Even though it is so automatic for me to reach for cigarettes in times of stress, I deeply and completely love and accept myself. I choose to consciously be aware of what I am doing so I can break this habit."

"Even though I need to smoke when the bills come in, I deeply and completely love and accept myself. I choose to change my behavior and put on the kettle or take a few deep breaths instead of smoking."

"Even though I have an intense urge to smoke when I'm stuck in traffic, I deeply and completely love and accept myself. I choose to forgive myself and anybody else involved and have the courage to resist this urge."

"Even though I must smoke before I speak to certain people to calm my nerves, I deeply and completely love and accept myself. I choose to easily and deliberately release my smoking need."

"Even though I must smoke at least a packet of cigarettes to get through all the extra work I take home with me, I deeply and completely love and accept myself. I choose instead to eat healthy snacks to give me the real energy to get through all the work I need to get done."

Myth #6 Smoking Gives Me Pleasure

Can you remember the very first time you smoked a cigarette? Can you honestly say it gave you great pleasure?

Most people claim they didn't enjoy their first few cigarettes. That's because the body rejects the poison that's inhaled.

It's likely that you would have told yourself it was pleasurable because others told you so.

The truth is, the pleasure in smoking is artificially induced by each cigarette approximately 30 minutes after smoking it.

Your mind tells you that you enjoy it. Your mind makes the association subconsciously with relief, fear and anxiety. And your mind makes a mythical association with relaxation, stress relief and sociability.

These are all sensations we would find enjoyable.

Luckily EFT easily dismisses this false illusion of enjoyment, and will make it easy for you to stop smoking.

While tapping on the following setup phrases, hold and look at a cigarette while imagining how enjoyable it would be to smoke it.

> "Even though I don't believe the truth about pleasure and smoking, I deeply and completely love and accept myself. I choose to accept that perhaps I'm not ready to stop smoking just yet."
>
> "Even though I will miss out on fun, pleasure and enjoyment if I stop smoking, I deeply and completely love and accept myself. I choose to accept that it is possible to have fun, pleasure and enjoyment without smoking."
>
> "Even though I really do enjoy smoking, I deeply and completely love and accept myself. I choose to understand that my mind falsely associates smoking with pleasure."

www.TheHiddenSecretsofEFT.com

"Even though I am killing myself quickly and prefer inhaling noxious gas rather than fresh air, I deeply and completely love and accept myself. I choose to face reality and remember the true taste of cigarettes when I first started smoking."

"Even though I associate the false sense of security smoking gives me with pleasure, I deeply and completely love and accept myself. I choose to use EFT to nurture my own security that is found only inside of me, and not within a cigarette."

Myth #7 Smoking Keeps Me Thin

Contrary to what many people believe, there isn't a direct correlation between giving up smoking and weight gain.

Stopping smoking and eating less, both advocate the use of willpower. As we've already discussed previously, willpower is not needed to give up smoking or to lose weight.

You may put on weight, only because you need to physically find a replacement for your smoking habit and you may need to do something with your hands. Food helps in both cases.

What you don't want to do is transfer your smoking addiction into an eating addiction. We want to heal the root cause of why you smoke—not keep the same problem and disguise it via over-eating.

Please be aware, that if you're looking for a new source of comfort, turning to food is an easy option (which is why you could end up over-eating). Eating or snacking every hour instead of smoking a cigarette is merely another crutch.

Those who stop smoking do not have a problem with food or over-eating. This is because they have healed the root problem, and their underlying addiction doesn't take on another guise.

If you find yourself over-eating, this may be a sign that you haven't healed the root problem.

Let's get to the real roots of the belief that smoking keeps you thin with these setup phrases...

"Even though I like the weight I am now and don't want to stop smoking because I'm scared I'll get fat, I deeply and completely love and accept myself. I choose to accept the fact I will only gain weight if I eat excessively."

"Even though there's no way I can maintain a healthy weight and stop smoking, I deeply and completely love and accept myself. I choose to be open to the possibility that perhaps I can stop smoking easily and remain thin."

"Even though I've cut down my cigarettes, but feel nervous and restless and want to turn to food, I deeply and completely love and accept myself. I choose to only eat when I am physically hungry."

"Even though I am over-eating to replace my cigarettes and I find comfort in this, I deeply and completely love and accept myself. I choose to let the real reason come up, and not eat just because I am emotionally hungry."

"Even though my intense craving for cigarettes has forced me into over-eating, I deeply and completely love and accept

myself. I choose to see my behavior for what it is—an emotional crutch, that still leaves the root problem unresolved."

Myth #8 My Cravings Are too Strong

Nicotine cravings are simply a voice inside your head telling you to smoke, that Richard Craze labels so well in his book, *The Voice of Tobacco*.

Craze speculates, that tobacco is merely a parasite that uses the human body (and mind) as a host. This assertion seems very accurate. Smoking offers no true benefits, only illusions of well-being.

Do you sleep perfectly well at night without sweating and becoming anxious, because of your nicotine craving? At a guess, you answered yes.

So why are you not able to go through the day for more than a couple of hours, without a cigarette?

The withdrawal from nicotine is the same as a withdrawal from any other drug, except that it is far milder. If you have given up in the past you will understand how frightening it is.

The cessation of smoking cigarettes promotes anxiety, and withdrawal causes restlessness, sweating, irritability, insomnia, nervousness and fatigue.

The artificial anxiety induced by smoking, will probably last about four days if allowed to decrease naturally within the body.

Unfortunately, you may smoke again within these 4 days. It's normal to feel the urge to smoke again, because you'll think that smoking will relieve your feelings of discomfort.

It's important you recognize this for what it is—another illusion.

Non-smoking partners of those who smoke, don't suffer withdrawal symptoms when their partner stops smoking.

They inhale the same nicotine (albeit passively). Yet because non-smoking partners don't have any negative emotional associations with smoking, they don't experience cravings.

Here are some setup phrases...

> "Even though I feel panicked at the thought of stopping smoking, I deeply and completely love and accept myself. I choose to allow myself to break free from the continuous cycle of anxiety that smoking keeps me in."
>
> "Even though I've heard about the withdrawal symptoms and I don't want to experience them (and therefore continuing to smoke), I deeply and completely love and accept myself. I choose to release any fear or nervousness I feel, one breath at a time."
>
> "Even though I feel like I'm going to die because the withdrawal symptoms are so bad, I deeply and completely love and accept myself. I choose to accept mild discomfort now, instead of dying young."
>
> "Even though I feel irritable, crabby and mad because I've just stopped smoking, I deeply and completely love and accept

myself. With grace and love I choose to express, rather than suppress my feelings."

"Even though I cannot sleep and I feel like I'm drowning in nerves, I deeply and completely love and accept myself. I choose to constructively distract myself, by reading a book or putting on a movie."

"Even though what I am experiencing now is excruciating and no one seems to understand what I'm going through, I deeply and completely love and accept myself. I choose to see things in perspective. Four days of discomfort now, in return for the rest of my life."

"Even though I am craving nicotine so desperately, I deeply and completely love and accept myself. I choose to realize that this feeling is temporary and will soon pass."

Case Study

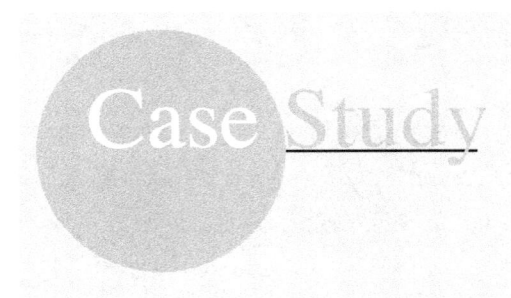

EFT was one of the most amazing tools for a client of mine that wanted to stop smoking.

Not only was he able to use EFT to cope with cravings, but also identified the real underlying issue that was connected to his smoking in the first place. He had been smoking since the age of 16 when his parents divorced.

We initially began by placing a cigarette on the table in front of him and scaled his craving between 0–10.

We started by tapping on the cravings he was having…

"Even though I have this craving for that cigarette, I love and accept myself anyway, and now choose to let that craving go."

"Even though I would still like to smoke that cigarette, I now choose to let those cravings go completely, and feel calm and relaxed instead."

I asked my client to focus on the idea of stopping his smoking habit and just notice what came to mind.

We tapped on…

> "Even though it makes me nervous to think about stopping my smoking, I love and accept myself anyway, and choose instead to feel confident in my ability to stop."
>
> "Even though part of me enjoys smoking and doesn't really want to stop smoking, I choose now to let that feeling go and remember how important it is for my health to quit."

And then we tapped on…

> "Even though I'm afraid I won't be able to deal with the physical cravings, I love and accept myself anyway. I now choose to feel calm and assured that I will easily be able to handle the cravings."

Once my client was able to feel comfortable with the idea of stopping, I asked him to think about the "upside of continuing to smoke" and the "downside of stopping to smoke," in order to identify more aspects that needed to be tapped on.

My client felt the upside of smoking, was being accepted by others that he smoked with on his work breaks.

He felt the downside of stopping, was dealing with anxious feelings underlying the smoking.

So we tapped on the following statements…

> "Even though I'm afraid that others at work will bother me if I stop, and tempt me to smoke, maybe I can choose to let that fear go and trust in my ability to say no to them."

"Even though I'm afraid others at work will reject me if I stop smoking—since we won't have that in common anymore, I love and accept myself anyway and choose to feel good about my decision to stop."

"Even though I don't think I can handle the anxious feelings underlying my smoking habit, I love and accept myself anyway. I now choose to find a healthy way to deal with my anxious feelings instead."

I then asked my client how long he had used smoking to cope with anxious feelings, and what exactly was going on in his life at age 16 when he started smoking.

He remembered that his parents were going through a divorce when he had his first cigarette at his friend's house. He had gone to his friend's house that day because he felt anxious when his parents were yelling and fighting about getting the divorce.

This was clearly the root of his smoking addiction. He had been using smoking for years to not feel the emotional pain and anxiety about his parents' divorce. So we tapped on…

"Even though I have used smoking to deal with my anxious feelings for such a long time, I love, accept and forgive myself fully and completely."

"Even though I'm afraid to feel all the emotions surrounding my parents' divorce, I love and accept myself anyway and I now choose to deal with those emotions in a healthy and safe way."

As I allowed my client to take a moment and identify how he felt that day his parents were fighting, and about the divorce overall, he was able to feel emotions of anxiety, sadness, grief, and guilt.

We then took the time to tap on each of them separately as follows…

> *"Even though I felt anxious about my parents fighting that day, I love and accept myself anyway, and now choose to let that anxious feeling go."*
>
> *"Even though I felt so sad when my parents decided to split up, I love and accept myself anyway, and now choose to let that sadness go so that I can be at peace."*
>
> *"Even though I have all this grief about my parents' divorce, I now choose to let that feeling go, and choose to begin seeing the situation in a more loving light."*
>
> *"Even though I have this guilty feeling—like my parents' divorce was somehow my fault—I love and accept myself anyway, fully and completely, trusting that their divorce was about them and not about me."*

It is quite common for all types of addictions to be connected to some sort of negative life event. When a person uses alcohol, drugs, gambling, smoking or work to escape from feeling any negative emotions, those emotions become repressed.

The individual then has to continue with the addiction, often using more and more, in order to not feel the underlying emotions.

From this example we can see that by asking the client what was going on in their life at the time they started using their addictive substance, can provide the answer to the root cause.

EFT can then be used to deal with all those emotions in a healthy way, so that the brain can let go of the event, and the individual can move forward with their life in a new way.

www.TheHiddenSecretsofEFT.com

www.TheHiddenSecretsofEFT.com

How to Upgrade Your Thoughts to Increase Your Bank Balance

"No one can become rich without enriching others. Anyone who adds to prosperity must prosper in turn."
~ G. Alexander Orndorff

www.TheHiddenSecretsofEFT.com

Increase Prosperity, Money and Abundance with EFT

It is true, that money alone cannot guarantee you happiness, but why do so many of us work long hours and strive to have more of it? Certainly more money can make your life easier, providing you more choice and ultimately more freedom.

We are often told that if we desire something enough, it will surely come to us. When the desired circumstance or thing doesn't arrive, we ask ourselves why not? What did we do (or not do) to prevent us receiving what we desire?

Few of us are happy with the amount of wealth and abundance in our lives.

It is likely that if what you desire isn't materializing in your life, it is because you have a strong negative emotional resistance.

There are so many variables as to why you are stopping, preventing and resisting more wealth coming into your life. For this reason, I've dedicated a lot of material to this important chapter.

The Importance of Money

Money is important. Money alone can impact, change and improve your life dramatically; therefore, it's vital we learn about and understand the true nature of money.

www.TheHiddenSecretsofEFT.com

Money is a form of energy and responds to you accordingly. For instance, if you treat money respectfully it will be attracted to you and want to stay with you. If you treat money badly, it will be repelled by you and not stay with you for long.

Have you ever told yourself, "Oh it is just money?" If so, you are playing down its value.

Have you ever seen a coin on the road and not bothered (or been embarrassed) to pick it up because, "it is only 5 cents?" If you don't value or respect 5 cents, it demonstrates you don't care much about money.

Please tap on the following setup statements…

> *"Even though I never believed money was important, I can love and accept myself anyway, fully and completely. I now choose to understand the amount of wealth in my life is a reflection of me."*

> *"Even though I tell myself over and over that 'it is just money', I can love and accept myself anyway, fully and completely. I now choose to be open to respecting money more."*

> *"Even though I place little value on small amounts of money, I can love and accept myself anyway, fully and completely. I now choose to cherish and look after all denominations of money, big or small."*

Growing Up in Lack

If at this present moment you don't have much money, you're most likely focusing on what you do not have.

It's nearly impossible to feel financially secure if you grew up in scarcity, and are most likely living in scarcity now.

Juggling bills, spending money before your paycheck arrives, or living off credit cards or other borrowed money, may be all too familiar to you.

Tap on the following setup phrases to dissolve any resentment you may still harbor as a result of growing up without wealth and abundance.

"Even though I resent the fact I grew up in a poor family that struggled to make ends meet, I can love and accept myself anyway, fully and completely. I now choose to understand my parents did the best they could."

"Even though I resent not having the opportunities the other kids did (such as going on an annual vacation), I can love and accept myself anyway, fully and completely. I now choose to forgive everyone involved."

"Even though I resent the fact I don't have a better paid job now, because my family couldn't afford to send me to university, I can love and accept myself anyway, fully and completely. I now choose to believe it is never too late for wealth to enter my life."

"Even though living in scarcity is all I know and am familiar with, I can love and accept myself anyway, fully and completely. I now choose to be open to living more abundantly with more wealth in my life."

"Even though there is never enough money and I am living in debt, I can love and accept myself anyway, fully and completely. I now choose to shift my attention to what I do have and not on what I don't have."

"Even though I resent the fact money goes out faster than it comes in, I can love and accept myself anyway, fully and completely. I now choose to believe that whatever money I have, is more than enough to cover all my outgoings."

"Even though my family never had money, and is why I don't have money, I can love and accept myself anyway, fully and completely. I now choose to accept that what happened in my past does not decide my future today."

Having a Limited Mind-set

For those people who are living in scarcity, it is likely they have a limited mind-set. There is a set amount of money each person is comfortable with.

How much are you comfortable earning each year? How many notes do you feel comfortable carrying in your purse at any one time? How much money can you own before others will resent you? You will find the amounts to be quite specific.

Essentially, we subconsciously limit the amount of money that comes into our lives. And if we come into possession of a large sum of money, we will quickly find a way to spend that money so we can feel comfortable again at our benchmark amount.

Tap on the following setup phrases to dissolve your discomfort surrounding money…

> *"Even though I am comfortable with X amount of money in my life and no more, I can love and accept myself anyway, fully and completely. I now choose to expand my comfort zone accepting more money into my life, easily and consistently."*

> *"Even though earning too much money would mean my friends and family wouldn't accept me, I can love and accept myself anyway, fully and completely. I now choose to accept that this belief is holding me back from allowing more abundance into my life."*

> *"Even though I feel uncomfortable handling, managing and accepting money, I can love and accept myself anyway, fully and completely. I now choose to learn about money so I can enjoy more of it in my life."*

Neutralizing Resentment

Although we may not like to admit it, many of us feel and speak negatively about those who have significantly more wealth than we do.

Resentment is a dangerous emotion if you harbor it, and it can keep wealth and abundance away from you.

If you actively dislike those who are wealthy (or whose lifestyles are synonymous with having money), then your subconscious mind will not allow you to become like these affluent people.

If you are jealous of, or resent people who have what you want (whatever that may be), then your subconscious mind will protect and prevent you from being the same as them.

If you would like to enjoy more wealth and abundance in your life, it is useful first to pinpoint any specific feelings of resentment you have.

Use the setup statements below as a guide to tap away any emotional resentment you have…

"Even though I don't like to admit feelings of jealousy or resentment of other's wealth, I can love and accept myself anyway, fully and completely. I now choose to be open and honest about any negative feelings I have, so I can deal with them once and for all."

"Even though it's not fair because I work harder than X, yet earn less money, I can love and accept myself anyway, fully and completely. I now choose to celebrate the wealth I do have, and not worry how much others make."

"Even though I begrudge the fact that X has access to private medicine and I don't, I can love and accept myself anyway, fully and completely. I now choose to understand that the things I resent, can never be attracted to me."

"Even though I'm jealous because X has a vacation home in Spain, and we can't even afford a weekend away, I can love and accept myself anyway, fully and completely. I now choose to believe that what is possible for others, is also possible for me too."

"Even though it is wrong for people to earn six figures or more each year, while the rest of us are struggling, I can love and accept myself anyway, fully and completely. I now choose to believe there is plenty of money for everyone to earn as much as they want."

"Even though I dislike people who are enjoying life and not working hard, I can love and accept myself anyway, fully and completely. I now choose to understand it's possible to work smart and enjoy life simultaneously."

Common Limiting Beliefs About Money

There are many beliefs surrounding money that we take on automatically without even questioning if the beliefs are true or not.

If a belief is not serving you, it is time to discard it and replace it with a more truthful one.

The setup statements below are examples of typical myths surrounding wealth, money and abundance. Please tap on them and any others that come to mind…

"Even though I resent rich people because I believe they are arrogant, greedy or rude, I can love and accept myself anyway, fully and completely. I now choose to understand that as long as I believe in this stereotype, I can never be rich myself."

"Even though it's impossible for me to make a lot of money as I was not well-educated, I can love and accept myself anyway, fully and completely. I now choose to understand that many of the wealthiest people in the world didn't even finish high school."

"Even though I despise wealthy people because they flaunt their money and no one likes a show-off, I can love and accept myself anyway, fully and completely. I now choose to be happy for other's wealth."

"Even though I believe if I make too much money, someone else will lose out, I can love and accept myself anyway, fully and completely. I now choose to accept the fact there is an unlimited supply of money in the world and plenty for everyone."

"Even though it is more spiritual to be poor than rich, I can love and accept myself anyway, fully and completely. I now choose to accept the more money I have, the more people I can help."

"Even though deep down I believe money is the root of all evil, I can love and accept myself anyway, fully and completely. I now choose to understand this statement was passed onto me by someone else, and I have a choice whether to believe it or not."

"Even though I believe life is meant to be a struggle because it's supposed to be character-building, I can love and accept myself anyway, fully and completely. I now choose to believe life can be free-flowing and easy if I allow it to be."

"Even though I believe with a passion that to be rich you must either be born into wealth or be extremely lucky, I can love and accept myself anyway, fully and completely. I now choose to look at the facts. Most of the people today who are rich created their own wealth and overcame exceptional circumstances."

How to Grow Your Money

Some people live and breathe money. Everything they do and every new idea they have, concerns the acquisition and retaining of money. Investments, stocks and bonds are the things they find exciting.

Have you ever heard the saying that "money goes to money?" There is truth in this, because those who are very wealthy (particularly the "nouveau riche") have invested wisely. In return, their investments have gained them rich returns.

To live in this world it costs money. We have to eat, wear clothes and keep a roof over our heads. The secret is in finding a balance in our finances that not only enables us to live comfortably, but have remaining money to work for us.

Please note, that an increase in income, does not necessarily mean an increase in wealth.

Typically when you earn more money, you will probably want to spend more. You may decide to upgrade your house and car, send your children to private schools or take longer and more expensive vacations.

www.TheHiddenSecretsofEFT.com

As a result, your accumulation of wealth is no greater. Although it may seem alien to you at first, it would be wise to familiarize yourself with and learn about investments. You can then decide where to invest future income, so your money can work for you.

Start the ball rolling by looking into the various investment opportunities available. Make a list of what you would like to achieve with your higher income.

Don't just list things that you can spend money on, but decide where you would like to be in five years' time. This will give you a much greater perspective.

An increase in wealth brings greater responsibility. This is one reason why many of us are scared to have enormous wealth. Doing something differently for the first time is scary. It's safer and easier to stay where we are, as familiarity is comfortable.

Please tap on the following setup phrases…

"Even though I am scared to have enormous wealth because of the increased responsibility, I can love and accept myself anyway, fully and completely. I now choose to be open to new responsibilities."

"Even though I don't have a clue how to look after, manage and grow my money, I can love and accept myself anyway, fully and completely. I now choose to seek financial help from an expert whose job it is to guide me."

"Even though I don't want to shoulder any responsibility to do

with wealth accumulation and retention (as I have too much responsibility with other things in my life), I can love and accept myself anyway, fully and completely. I now choose to take one step at a time, knowing I don't have to learn everything at once."

"Even though it is safe, comfortable and familiar to stay where I am financially, I can love and accept myself anyway, fully and completely. I now choose to accept that if I really want greater wealth in my life, I will have to embrace new ways of doing things."

"Even though money markets, investments and stocks are for other people and definitely not for me, I can love and accept myself anyway, fully and completely. I now choose to be open to learning about money."

"Even though I am frightened of money, I can love and accept myself anyway, fully and completely. I now choose to view money as being like a good friendship—something to be respected, cherished and nurtured."

"Even though I want to stay in my comfort zone, I can love and accept myself anyway, fully and completely. I now choose to be willing to slowly and deliberately stretch myself."

Are You Allergic To Money?

Sensitivities, intolerances and allergies are common place in our lives today. We can be allergic to any substance... certain foods, chemicals, smells, fabrics or dust, and money is no exception.

Would you be surprised to learn that most of us are allergic to money?

It can sometimes be difficult to find out why you may be sensitive towards money. Sometimes an allergy or sensitivity can occur, because of an emotion being incorrectly associated with a particular substance.

See if you can pinpoint a time when your wealth took a nosedive and determine what emotions were predominant during that time. Are there any correlations with your sensitivity to money today?

If so, then use EFT to clear any emotions that have been wrongly associated with money...

> "Even though I am weak and uncomfortable around money, I can love and accept myself anyway, fully and completely. I now choose to be open to finding out the root cause."
>
> "Even though I started to feel really uncomfortable around money when _____ happened, I can love and accept myself anyway, fully and completely. I now choose to be open to healing my discomfort around money."
>
> "Even though I have wrongly associated person X/incident with being uncomfortable around money, I can love and accept myself anyway, fully and completely. I now choose to see that person X/incident has nothing to do with money."
>
> "Even though I feel guilty/ashamed/confused because I have wrongly associated person X/incident with being uncomfortable around money, I can love and accept myself

anyway, fully and completely. I now choose to release and be free from any negative emotions now."

You can use Muscle Testing to determine if you are visibly weak around money. You will be able to determine the exact amount of money that makes you feel uncomfortable.

Once you know the amount of money that brings on discomfort, you can tap on this amount and then gradually raise the amount of money you feel comfortable with.

A lot of people think their salary reflects the amount of money they are worth.

If you feel you are only worth a certain amount, tap on why you think that is, and then use EFT to gradually raise the amount of money you feel you are really worth.

Tap on the following setup phrases...

> "Even though I feel uncomfortable around sums of money that exceed X amount, I can love and accept myself anyway, fully and completely. I now choose to dissolve any discomfort surrounding this specific amount."
>
> "Even though I feel uncomfortable around X amount of money, or more because _____ happened, I can love and accept myself anyway, fully and completely. I now choose to see that I've incorrectly associated the two."
>
> "Even though I'm unhappy with my salary (as I know I'm worth more), I can love and accept myself anyway, fully and completely. I now choose jobs with salaries to match what I know I am really worth."

www.TheHiddenSecretsofEFT.com

"Even though I feel greedy for wanting to have more money, I can love and accept myself anyway, fully and completely. I now choose to see that belief is limiting and restricting my wealth."

"Even though I feel I am only worth X amount of money each year, I can love and accept myself anyway, fully and completely. I now choose to raise the amount I'm worth, slowly but surely."

You Are Worthy

There have probably been many moments in your life when you felt you "weren't good enough" or deserving enough to live the life you desired.

These thoughts, self-limiting feelings and beliefs have probably been in your subconscious mind for many years. They were likely planted there due to what you heard while you were growing up.

We have all experienced statements and comments that never held any truth, yet we believed in them anyway.

Can you remember any comments around money, being told to you during your childhood that you can still remember today? Some comments may not have been spoken in malice, but have still impacted your life in some way.

What comments made you feel left out? What unkind names were you called? What did someone say to you that made you feel humiliated? Was there someone who made you feel useless, no good or worthless? What were you criticized for? Did you ever feel rejected and if so, why?

It's useful to understand that hurtful comments (whether intentional or not) may have had a destructive impact on your life.

As hard as it may be to accept, what you've been told does not necessarily define who you are today. Please create your own setup phrases using the following as examples…

"Even though Sam from school, told me I was useless at sports and would always pick me last for his team (leaving me feeling humiliated), I can love and accept myself anyway, fully and completely. I now choose to forgive Sam as it was just his opinion and not the truth."

"Even though Tania didn't let me play with her and I felt so left out and alone, I can love and accept myself anyway, fully and completely. I now choose to forgive Tania, maybe she was just a bossy girl."

"Even though I overheard my teacher telling another teacher that I was "the slow one", I can love and accept myself anyway, fully and completely. I now choose to forgive my teacher and not let her opinion define me."

"Even though dad told me that I had no talent in art, I can love and accept myself anyway, fully and completely. I now choose to forgive my Dad and understand that he came from a family where he was never praised, and negativity is all he knows."

"Even though my careers advisor said I'd only get low paid work with my qualifications, I can love and accept myself anyway, fully and completely. I now choose to see the truth, that qualifications don't necessarily equate to a high income."

"Even though so many people have said hurtful comments to me and I can't help them impacting my life, I can love and accept myself anyway, fully and completely. I now choose to forgive anyone involved and put myself first, and not listen to other's opinions of me."

Abundance Surrounds You

If you live in the Western hemisphere, then it is likely you already experience abundance in your life.

As human beings, we are constantly being challenged to reach further and attain more. It is the natural progression in life to be "more".

If you look around your current space, you can probably see you are already blessed with abundance. Depending on your experiences, you can change your mind-set from day-to-day about whether you feel "lucky" or not.

This is a great exercise in being more conscious and aware of what's around you.

What do you see? Do you see scarcity?

In each area of your life, do you see holes where your basic needs are not being met? Do you wish you had more?

Unfortunately, if you focus on the lack in your life, then this is what your life will continue to produce for you.

Do you see the bare essentials? Do you have a functional car but dream of a different model? Do you have food to survive, but little left over for luxuries? Do you own clothes, but wish you were better dressed? Do you have a roof over your head, but wish you had a flasher home?

If you focus only on having the bare minimum, then you will never accumulate what you truly desire.

Do you see great abundance? Do you feel gratitude that you've attained the things you desire for your family? Are you happy and satisfied with the level of wealth that you have achieved?

Luckily, if your focus is on the abundance around you and you acknowledge the great privileges in your life, then you will continue to generate more of the same.

In the Western world, we have had great abundance bestowed on us.

Every human being who resides on planet earth has been given air to breathe. We have been given air to fill our lungs which allow us to live. We should acknowledge and feel grateful for this.

In our Western society we have water on tap. How amazing that we can go to any tap in the house, simply turn on a valve and there is water. We could not survive without it, and the universe supplies this for us in abundance.

In countries where water is scarce, there are immense problems in the infrastructure, as well as people dying from the lack of it.

One third of the planet's population do not have enough to eat. In our Western society we have supermarkets and malls brimming over with food abundance. The choice is mind boggling. And in the wild, we can find fruit, berries and wild herbs.

We take all of this for granted, but if it was suddenly taken away from us, it would only be then that we'd realize just how full of abundance our lives had really been.

The chain of abundance begins with the tiny wheat seed that the farmer plants in the ground. He grows the wheat for us so we can have bread. The dairy herdsman looks after his cows so we can have milk.

To change your mind-set from lack to abundance, all you need to do is "count your blessings." Be grateful that you can put food on the table, house your family and put clothes on your back. Being able to enjoy family life together is abundance indeed.

Bless and give thanks for the abundance that you have throughout your day–from waking in the morning to retiring at night, your journey to work, your ability to work and the food you eat throughout your day.

Give thanks to the friendly man at the news stand who greets you every morning, the coffee shop that sells your favorite coffee to kick-start your day, your coworkers, your boss and your paycheck at the end of the working month.

Be grateful for your safe return home at the end of the day and your family who greets you. Give thanks to your crying baby who is healthy and growing. Give thanks...

All of these events are abundances in your life. Count your blessings and give thanks!

Tap on the following setup phrase...

> *"Even though I have not been fully aware of the infinite abundance which surrounds me, I can love and accept myself anyway, fully and completely. I now choose to forgive myself, and experience the complete abundance which surrounds me in all areas of my life."*

Changing Your Attitude to Gratitude

When you complain about everything that is happening in your life, or your perceived lack of abundance, it can quickly turn into a bad habit.

Do you complain about having to get up in the morning? Do you complain about the traffic when traveling to work?

Do you complain that your boss over-works and under-pays you? Do you gossip about a misdemeanor that someone has done to somebody else? Do you fuel rumors by spreading comments about what you have heard about X?

All of the above creates an atmosphere of negativity and ungratefulness in general, that will shape your life.

If you continually find fault with everything and everyone in your life, the energy that flows back to you will return as similar negativity.

On the contrary, finding gratitude in every moment may be a sea of change in the behavior you are currently practising. It is imperative to your own personal well-being that you actively seek out, and be thankful for everything and everyone in your life.

As a society we are materialistic and critical. We are quick to complain about something. We find it more difficult to show gratitude and thanks.

Think about all the people you know. The happy, joyful ones stand out a mile, because most people simply are not like this.

This is not to say that you are forbidden to express your emotions through dark periods in your life. It can be difficult to feel positive thoughts or feelings when we are deeply unhappy about something.

In every perceived negative event in your life, a lesson can be learnt from it.

Other people may have caused you pain. Perhaps a close friend has let you down in some way. Perhaps you have experienced a divorce or have a serious problem with one of your children. Maybe you are unwell or dying.

It is normal and natural to express emotions of anger, frustration, sadness and sorrow. It is not normal however, or healthy, to harbor these feelings indefinitely.

If bitterness, disappointment or any other negative emotion stays with you in your life, now is the time to release them.

You can show appreciation and gratitude for your life now, yet still desire something different.

Please tap on the following setup phrases…

"Even though I have complained about everything in my life, I can love and accept myself anyway, fully and completely. I now choose to focus on all wonderful things in my life that I have neglected to notice."

"Even though I have unknowingly created a negative outlook on my life, I can love and accept myself anyway, fully and completely. I now choose to change my mind-set towards gratitude."

"Even though I have been quick to complain, criticize and gossip, I can love and accept myself anyway, fully and completely. I now choose to praise, appreciate, and keep silent when I can't say anything positive."

"Even though _____ event occurred in my past and I just can't leave my sadness/disappointment/anger behind, I can love and accept myself anyway, fully and completely. I now choose to release my emotions so they don't cloud my life today."

"Even though I don't know how to express and/or release my negativity, I can love and accept myself anyway, fully and completely. I now choose to trust in the process of EFT to free myself from emotional pain."

Directing Your Focus

All of us receive what we focus on. There are no exceptions to this Universal Law which applies to everything and everyone.

If you are focusing on your perceived lack of abundance, then you will receive a lack of abundance. If you show gratitude for what you have, then you will receive more of what you are grateful for.

Whatever attitude you are giving out, is the one you receive back into your life. The Universe will simply reflect everything that you are focusing on.

If this concept is difficult for you to accept, please tap on the following setup phrases…

"Even though I don't believe it is true that what I focus on manifests in my life, I can love and accept myself anyway, fully and completely. I now choose to be open to seeing the truth."

"Even though I think positive thoughts but bad things still happen to me (so it can't be true that what I focus on turns up in my life), I can love and accept myself anyway, fully and completely. I now choose to accept the fact that I must be

www.TheHiddenSecretsofEFT.com

focusing more on bad things than good. I actively change my focus."

It's true that it's difficult to change your way of thinking as you are accustomed to reacting and behaving in a certain manner. Yet, if you would like to see different opportunities and more abundance in your life you must do this...

Tap on the following setup phrases...

"Even though I can't possibly change the way I've always thought, I can love and accept myself anyway, fully and completely. I now choose to be open to slowly and consciously choosing different thoughts."

"Even though I have so many negative thoughts, I don't know where to start, and I feel overwhelmed, I can love and accept myself anyway, fully and completely. I now choose to tackle one thought at a time. There is no rush."

You can begin by removing the negative thoughts and feelings about what you think you don't have.

The setup phrases listed below are examples of common grumbles. Please add your own grievance if it is not listed below, and tap until the statement no longer produces negative emotions in you.

"Even though I don't have a well-paid job, I can love and accept myself anyway, fully and completely. I now choose to be grateful that I even have a job, and feel lucky I am employed."

"Even though I don't have a job I enjoy, I can love and accept myself anyway, fully and completely. I now choose to find joy in the job I have or seek something different."

"Even though I didn't have a good education, I can love and accept myself anyway, fully and completely. I now choose to let this fact not influence me, or return to study."

"Even though I am not good-looking enough/too fat/too ugly, I can love and accept myself anyway, fully and completely. I now choose to accept myself for who I am, knowing I have the freedom to make any positive lifestyle changes I wish."

"Even though I lack confidence in myself, I can love and accept myself anyway, fully and completely. I now choose to be open in increasing my confidence more each day, building it slowly."

"Even though I don't have any friends, I can love and accept myself anyway, fully and completely. I now choose to accept myself completely, knowing that when I do this, others too will accept me."

"Even though I am unfit but can't afford to go to my local gym, I can love and accept myself anyway, fully and completely. I now choose to stop making excuses. Walking is free."

"Even though I feel like a failure as I am not in a romantic relationship or married, I can love and accept myself anyway, fully and completely. I now choose to love myself… because only when I love myself, can others love me."

"Even though I don't have enough money to pay my bills and

I am sinking further into debt, I can love and accept myself anyway, fully and completely. I now choose to do something practical and take control of my financial situation."

"Even though I don't have a top of the range car, I can love and accept myself anyway, fully and completely. I now choose to think of ways I can generate more money to save towards my dream car."

"Even though I don't own my own home and the house I'm renting is a dump, I can love and accept myself anyway, fully and completely. I now choose to be grateful for the roof I have over my head, and trust that the home I'd like to own one day can be a reality for me."

Now that you've made peace with your common "gripes" it's time to be grateful and appreciative for the blessings already in your life.

Please make a list including all the seemingly "small things." Things, like your favorite song playing on the radio, the birds singing or the rain falling. Aim for at least 100 things on your list.

Here are some examples to get you started:

- I can borrow books free from the library
- I have perfect vision
- I have full use of my body
- I can have a hot bath with scented candles at the end of a busy day
- I have an income that provides me with things I need

www.TheHiddenSecretsofEFT.com

- I have a loving child
- I have a close friend that I can rely on, no matter what
- I have the freedom to change myself
- I have the opportunity to learn whatever I want
- I can go for a walk whenever I like
- I have a garden that I love
- I can change things in my life today, which will create a better tomorrow
- I am alive
- I have food in my cupboard
- I have a car that works

Whenever you think of something else, add that to your list too. When you feel challenged about your attitude and feel tempted to complain, retrieve your list and read it through. It will automatically shift your focus and lift your spirits.

You can also tap on the following setup phrases…

"Even though I have been discontented with all the things I don't have, I can love and accept myself anyway, fully and completely. I now choose to be grateful for all the things on my list."

"Even though I have had difficulty in seeing the existing abundance in my life, because I've been so focused on what I don't have, I can love and accept myself anyway, fully and completely. I now choose to forgive myself and fill my life with an attitude of gratitude for all I already have."

Throughout your day, be on the lookout for things you can be grateful for. Awareness is the key here.

Some days you will be challenged by something that happens to you, and you'll be tempted to think negatively. At these times, focus on the good in the bad—stop, affirm and tap.

When you actively create a state of mind that doesn't become overcrowded with ungrateful thoughts and negative emotions, you will soon become a positive person everyone will want to be around.

And when you are grateful for the beauty that surrounds you and for the love of the people in your life, more beauty and more love will come into your life.

Learning to Give (and Enjoying It)

How willingly do you give to others?

In society, we are so intent on the attainment of material things or status, that we can forget how joyous it is to give something to someone else.

Yet, every year we demonstrate our need for giving, when millions of us give to charity telethons that are organized in almost every country in the world. (Even when our economy is suffering, this kind of fund-raising still creates millions of dollars for worthy charities.)

So what does this say about us?

Generally, human beings are motivated by the plights of others to do "their bit". Many people give to charities year round, some allotting a percentage of their monthly salaries to their favorite charity.

Why are some people able to do this while others are not?

If you were raised in an atmosphere of scarcity, then scarcity would likely be permeating your life today. You believe that you barely have enough for yourself; therefore, giving to someone else means you will probably go without.

When you give unconditionally (with the certainty the Universe will provide for you), this act of trust creates space in your life for even more abundance and wealth to enter.

This is worth repeating. *The act of giving creates the space in your life for more abundance to enter.*

Please tap on the following setup phrases...

"Even though I have no money to donate to charities I believe in, I can love and accept myself anyway, fully and completely. I now choose to open my mind to the possibility that I don't have to give money, I can give my time. Giving is giving."

"Even though I don't want to give my time or money, as I don't have enough of either, I can love and accept myself anyway, fully and completely. I now choose to make time or allocate money, to supporting those I care about."

"Even though I simply don't trust that if I give money away that it will be returned to me in some way, I can love and accept myself anyway, fully and completely. I now choose to

suspend this belief and try this law for myself before passing judgement."

Think of all the people that you love and who love you. Think of the small child who brings such joy into your life, the friend who is there for you in times of uncertainty and the partner who loves you unconditionally.

You are being given to, every day!

Even when you are given something small (such as a smile), be grateful and be willing to give something back—without question or counting the cost.

What emotions come up for you when you think about giving without expecting anything in return?

Turn these emotions into setup phrases and tap on any conflicting emotions.

For example…

> *"Even though the thought of giving something in return for nothing is alien to me, I can love and accept myself anyway, fully and completely. I now choose to be open to giving without any expectations."*
>
> *"Even though it is not in my character to give something for nothing and I would feel silly, I can love and accept myself anyway, fully and completely. I now choose to step outside my normal behavior and try it anyway."*
>
> *"Even though I have nothing to give, I can love and accept myself anyway, fully and completely. I now choose to think*

outside the square. I can give my time, my talents and my love."

"Even though I only like to give because I expect something in return, I can love and accept myself anyway, fully and completely. I now choose to practice giving for the sheer joy of it without any hidden agenda."

If you have been raised in an atmosphere of scarcity or lack, now is the time to clear this baggage.

Please tap on the following setup phrases. If any other negative feelings about giving emerge, clear them as you go with EFT.

"Even though I never have enough, I can love and accept myself anyway, fully and completely. I now choose to be open to the fact I have more than enough."

"Even though I have so little money and I cannot afford to give any away, I can love and accept myself anyway, fully and completely. I now choose to trust that all my immediate needs will be met fully and easily."

"Even though I don't have time to give to others, I can love and accept myself anyway, fully and completely. I now choose to dissolve this limiting belief. I have the same amount of time as everyone else in the world."

"Even though I have difficulty being generous to those I don't know, I can love and accept myself anyway, fully and completely. I now choose to practice giving to all kinds of people until this becomes second nature to me."

"Even though I find it hard to share love with others, I can love and accept myself anyway, fully and completely. I now choose to forgive myself and do the best I can."

"Even though I only live to give to those who deserve it and not to people who already have plenty of money, I can love and accept myself anyway, fully and completely. I now choose to give to everyone and not just those who are worse off than me."

"Even though I find it hard to give my time, money and love freely without condition or expectation, I can love and accept myself anyway, fully and completely. I now forgive myself and choose to be more generous and kind every day."

Learning to Receive

Learning to give freely with joy (and without counting the cost) is a huge step in our self-development. Once we've mastered this, the next step is learning to receive.

As hard as it may be for us to give, it'll probably be harder for us to receive—especially with grace and dignity.

Many of us have been raised with beliefs that it's not good to accept things from strangers, or that we shouldn't take more than we deserve.

This has left us with energy patterns which have lead us to believe we are not deserving of "more than our fair share." Or that if we take something, there won't be enough left for others.

www.TheHiddenSecretsofEFT.com

This leaves us with a moral dilemma of how much is your share, and what share do you personally deserve?

Before we go further, please tap on the following setup phrases…

> *"Even though I don't feel comfortable receiving things from others, I can love and accept myself anyway, fully and completely. I now choose to accept that a heartfelt "thank-you" is all that is needed when I am given something."*
>
> *"Even though I was taught not to accept things from other people unless it was my birthday or Christmas, I can love and accept myself anyway, fully and completely. I now choose to practice receiving with thanks, anything, at any time."*
>
> *"Even though I am annoyed when someone gets me something and I haven't gotten them anything in return, I can love and accept myself anyway, fully and completely. I now choose to understand that there is no score-keeping when it comes to gratitude."*
>
> *"Even though I have been brought up to believe it is greedy to accept something from someone else, I can love and accept myself anyway, fully and completely. I now choose to understand that it makes the person happy when giving. I choose to receive, instead of deny what they are giving."*
>
> *"Even though I am in the habit of saying "you shouldn't have" or, "you didn't have to do that," I can love and accept myself anyway, fully and completely. I now choose to accept with gratitude and love what has been bestowed on me."*

The Universe provides enough to go around for all of us. Abundance will come to us through no effort on our part. Or we may have worked extremely hard to provide a desirable life for ourselves or our family.

Sometimes, we may have a benefactor who wants to ease our way. Some may acknowledge and welcome this, others may not enjoy the fact that they received something they have not worked for or feel they deserve.

We covered earlier the topic of joy that we can feel when we give freely to others, believing that the Universe will provide us with everything that we need.

Therefore, the other side of receiving is allowing others to give. We must allow others to experience the same joy, when giving to us.

This will allow the energy of abundance to flow freely from one to another. By accepting a gift someone wishes to give, we allow them the joy and pleasure of giving.

Please tap on the following setup phrases...

> *"Even though I don't like the idea of being handed abundance without me working hard for it, I can love and accept myself anyway, fully and completely. I now choose to gratefully receive abundance in all forms."*
>
> *"Even though I will only accept wealth into my life if I feel I deserve it, I can love and accept myself anyway, fully and completely. I now choose to gratefully receive abundance in all forms."*

www.TheHiddenSecretsofEFT.com

"Even though I have taken away the joy of others by refusing what they are giving, I can love and accept myself anyway, fully and completely. I now choose to give others the joy of giving, by accepting what they offer with grace."

"Even though I have denied wealth and abundance into my life time and time again, I can love and accept myself anyway, fully and completely. I now choose to welcome it with open arms."

"Even though I believe we should give and not take, I can love and accept myself anyway, fully and completely. I now choose to give and receive with love and gratitude."

An unhealthy view of money can lead to all kinds of problems, both financial and emotional. If you have difficulty accepting the gifts that the Universe provides, then you will encourage periods of scarcity in your life.

Please tap on the following setup statements…

"Even though I don't allow money into my life, I can love and accept myself anyway, fully and completely. I now choose to be open to accepting wealth and abundance into my life in any form."

"Even though I accept money into my life but spend it as quickly as I can, I can love and accept myself anyway, fully and completely. I now choose to be comfortable with money and allow it to stay with me."

"Even though I have hoarded money and been unable to enjoy the pleasure of spending it on myself or others, I can

love and accept myself anyway, fully and completely. I now choose to accept the fact that money can provide immense enjoyment."

"Even though I have refused gifts (believing I was doing the right thing), I can love and accept myself anyway, fully and completely. I now choose to gratefully accept the flow of wealth and abundance into my life now."

Recognizing Opportunities

There are many opportunities available to us in life. Some are presented to us clearly. We can see the way forward in our lives before us, especially if we are open to new things.

However, many opportunities arrive cloaked by something else, especially when our mind is closed and all we see are problems instead of a chance for change.

Recently, how often have you seen an opportunity to make your life better—perhaps one to increase your fitness, embark on a new relationship or begin a new business venture?

All of this is possible for you. It is abundant in the Universe and is available to you every day. Not just one opportunity, but many. Some opportunities will have been created by you or may simply pop up in front of you.

It is up to you to recognize an opportunity when you see one and decide whether to act upon it or not. But sometimes something is blocking us from taking action, even when we want to.

It is your subconscious mind that will dictate whether we are open to receiving and making the most of opportunities. Taking your destiny into your own hands is within all of us.

But if your subconscious mind makes the decision to react in the usual programmed way, you will remain stuck in your comfort zones and belief systems that you are accustomed to. Please tap on the following setup phrases...

> "Even though I have been unable to see the multiple opportunities in front of me, I can love and accept myself anyway, fully and completely. I now choose to actively look for and create my own."

> "Even though I have noticed opportunities in my life but passed so many of them by, I can love and accept myself anyway, fully and completely. I now choose to act on the next one that comes my way."

> "Even though I have only seen the negative side of everything, I can love and accept myself anyway, fully and completely. I now choose to see the good in the bad."

> "Even though my subconscious mind has kept me stuck in familiarity and the same patterns of thinking, I can love and accept myself anyway, fully and completely. I now choose to dissolve any beliefs that don't serve me and step into a new way of thinking."

Have you ever resisted an opportunity that you knew deep down inside was right for you? Perhaps the fear was too overpowering and left you unable to act.

Here are a few examples of everyday opportunities that have been there for the taking, but may have passed up. Please tap on the following setup phrases and add your own...

"Even though a relationship that I've always dreamed of has presented itself to me and I said no, I can love and accept myself anyway, fully and completely. I now choose to say yes to happiness next time around."

"Even though a business opportunity landed in my lap that was certain to increase my income (and I rejected it immediately), I can love and accept myself anyway, fully and completely. I now choose to take advantage of future chances for increased wealth and abundance."

"Even though I turned down the chance to travel to somewhere I've always wanted to go, I can love and accept myself anyway, fully and completely. I now choose to swallow my fears and say yes."

Perhaps you are so busy solving your current problems, that you don't see the abundant opportunities that surround you. Please tap on the following setup phrases...

"Even though I find it so difficult to see the opportunities that are either handed to me on a silver platter or disguised as hard work, I can love and accept myself anyway, fully and completely. I now choose to forgive myself, choosing to be more aware of the abundance surrounding me."

"Even though I'd rather make excuses for my situation than take personal responsibility, I can love and accept myself

anyway, fully and completely. I now choose to take decisive action when an appropriate opportunity next appears."

"Even though I have not seen or created the opportunities that could maximize my potential, I can love and accept myself anyway, fully and completely. I now choose to forgive myself, choosing to see, create and act upon all future opportunities."

Asking the Right Questions

Asking the right questions of ourselves will give us opportunities for greater expansion and freedom.

With the myriad of limiting beliefs that we all hold within us, we are setting ourselves up to fail.

Finding the correct opportunities to develop our lives, both personally and otherwise, is already a difficult task because of the limitations we put on ourselves. Are we doomed for failure?

By opening ourselves to all the possibilities around us, we can achieve increased abundance and wealth. The way in which we phrase the questions we ask ourselves, can be the route to much greater achievements.

For example, instead of stating that you can't afford it, ask yourself "how can I afford it?" When you state that you can't afford something, you shut down your thinking and any other possibilities entering.

When you ask yourself how you *can* afford something, the door opens for solutions and opportunities.

The Universe works in mysterious ways, giving you something that you may have asked for in a different shape or form.

For instance, you may have needed (and asked the Universe) for some extra money for your child's school fees without having to work harder. Rather than increasing your work hours, you received an unexpectedly generous tax return just in time to pay the school fees.

Maybe somebody gave you free tickets to a show you really wanted to see, rather than forking out $200.

Expand your abundance by developing different ways to ask the question. And be open to what the Universe may provide.

For example, you could ask yourself, what is the easiest and quickest way I can afford this? This question makes the assumption that there is not only a way for you to take advantage of the opportunity, but more than one way.

This increases your chances of making the correct decision for your future abundance. Choosing to open the door to questions such as this, provides further empowerment when considering your future actions.

Please tap on the following setup phrases…

"Even though I have closed my mind to future possibilities, I can love and accept myself anyway, fully and completely. I now choose to forgive myself, and focus on asking myself open-ended questions that force my mind to look for solutions."

"Even though I have been negative in my statements to myself, I can love and accept myself anyway, fully and completely. I now choose to ask myself how I can achieve the result I desire, instead of automatically thinking there is no hope."

"Even though I have missed out on multiple opportunities by neglecting to ask myself empowering questions, I can love and accept myself anyway, fully and completely. I now choose to be grateful. I can now open up my future to endless possibilities."

"Even though I have focused all my energy on not being able to do things, I can love and accept myself anyway, fully and completely. I now choose to ban limiting phrases such as, "I can't" from my vocabulary for good."

Here are some examples of open-ended questions that you may like the answer to. Please tap on any negative self-talk or limiting beliefs that pop up, as soon as your mind has supplied you with an answer.

- What small actions can I take today to make my dream come true?
- How can I find a way to send my child to private school?
- How can I find a way to take my family on vacation?

- What can I do to improve my situation at work?
- What steps can I take today to enjoy a healthier body?
- What can I do right now to improve my feelings of low self-esteem?
- What actions can I take to help me reach my goals?

Please tap on the following setup phrase…

"Even though I have not created opportunities that can maximize my potential, I can love and accept myself anyway, fully and completely. I now choose to easily and consistently see, create and act upon every opportunity that leads me closer towards my goals."

Creating and Reaching Your Goals

When asked what we want for our lives, we often find it easier to say what we *don't want*. If asked to recite what our goals are, most of us wouldn't be able to, or even list what we would like our achievements to be.

Many of us go through life not having any clear view of what we really want to experience.

Or if we do have goals, they are very generic; such as, a bigger house, nicer car or more money. These answers are too vague to put into action—to change these dreams into reality.

To achieve real and tangible abundance, or to realize your

dreams, it is imperative that you are very specific about what you hope to achieve.

Please tap on the following setup phrases…

"Even though I have not been clear before on what I have really wanted, I can love and accept myself anyway, fully and completely. I now choose to form a detailed idea of what I really want."

"Even though I have focused primarily on what I don't want, I can love and accept myself anyway, fully and completely. I now choose to shift my focus to what I do desire."

"Even though I have not spent much time thinking about what I'd like to achieve in my life, I can love and accept myself anyway, fully and completely. I now choose to accept that what I focus on will become my reality. I will now take the time and care into focusing on living a life I am proud of."

"Even though I had goals that were too generic and wishy-washy, I can love and accept myself anyway, fully and completely. I now choose goals that are filled with detail, specifics and desired achievement dates."

It has been shown that writing down your goals means that you are 80% more likely to achieve them, than if you don't. Think deeply about your desires. What would you like for your personal life?

Indulge in your wildest dreams. Enjoy yourself. No matter what you crave, there is no limit on what you can achieve.

Aim high. Be motivated about your deepest desires and look forward to achieving and enjoying them.

It's not necessary for you to know exactly how you will achieve your heart's desires. Just be sure about what they are, and be focused on attaining them.

For the Universe to provide for you, it needs to know what you want and you must feel comfortable asking for it.

It is your right as a human being to ask for your desires without limitations. Be confident and trust—ask in the right way and you will receive it. Remember that the Universe wishes to provide for you, but you have to help do its job.

We have all heard of "visualizing" before. This is where you have a very clear view of the thing or circumstance that you are aiming for in your mind.

An essential first step is that you decide upon what you want or need, and picture it vividly in your mind's eye.

Let's assume for now that you would like a bigger house in a more upmarket area. Sit quietly, close your eyes and "see" it clearly.

Are you seeing a modern apartment, detached period house or a house you've constructed yourself? How many bedrooms and levels does it have?

What color is the paint inside on the walls? What type of gardens do you have? How will you decorate the interior?

Once you have a clear picture of your ideal house, picture yourself living inside it. Include other members of your family who will be living in the house with you too and any pets.

See yourself waking up in your dream bed, inside your dream bedroom, in your dream home, in your dream neighborhood.

Go about your normal day eating breakfast and all the usual things you would do while you are at home. This makes your visualization more real and tangible.

You can also make a story board with the vision that you wish to achieve. You can either cut pictures from magazines, create screen-saver images that rotate on your computer, or draw the home or goal you would like on paper.

Have your story board in a visible position, so you can view it whenever you wish. Tap on any resistance that comes up for you while you are looking at your images.

It is important you remove any limiting beliefs surrounding your dreams being unachievable.

Please tap on the following setup phrases…

> *"Even though I feel silly indulging in my wildest dreams as I don't see the point—as they're not going to happen, I can love and accept myself anyway, fully and completely. I now choose to suspend disbelief and aim for what I truly want."*

"Even though I don't know how it's possible for my goals to manifest, I can love and accept myself anyway, fully and completely. I now choose to accept that I don't have to know how things will happen, I just have to be clear on what."

"Even though I feel guilty asking for what I really desire, and am only comfortable asking for what I think I'm deserving of, I can love and accept myself anyway, fully and completely. I now choose to forgive myself for harboring this self-limiting belief."

"Even though visualization is for new-age types and that's definitely not me, I can love and accept myself anyway, fully and completely. I now choose to accept that having a clear goal in mind is not "esoteric".

The Journey to Short-Term Goals

On your journey in manifesting your true desires, you will need to acknowledge smaller goals that will take you to your deepest desire of abundance. Each journey begins with one small step.

It will be easier for you to achieve your ultimate goal by breaking the journey down into manageable steps that you can achieve. Setbacks can be limiting and frustrating, and will tempt you to give up.

But if you keep reaching small goals, you will know that you're well on your way to achieving your target goal.

www.TheHiddenSecretsofEFT.com

For example, if you want to be a veterinary surgeon, this cannot happen overnight as the training and qualifications required, take time.

Perhaps you first need to find out where you can study and if there is an exam to sit to enter the university you wish to study at. You will need to find out how long it will likely take to finish your training.

Do you need emotional support from your family? Will you need financial help, and if so, do you need a loan?

Turn all the necessary steps into small goals and then set about taking action today. Some stages may need to be broken down even further to create even more easily attainable goals.

Keeping a diary of your journey to your goal is useful. Any negative self talk or emotional resistance can be tapped on, if it arises.

When you finally reach your goal, thank the Universe for enabling you to claim what is rightfully yours, and for helping you achieve your quest.

Shift Your Comfort Zones

Your own comfort zone is just that… comfortable—a place that is secure, warm and familiar—and we don't want to change it.

The problem with comfort zones is that they are limiting and they don't last forever, even if it feels as if your zone is permanent.

Here is a client as an example, Mandy. She had found a job she loved. As soon as she walked into the building, she knew for certain that this was the place for her. Her interview went well, and she really connected with the interviewer—the person who subsequently became her boss.

For six months, everything went well. Mandy was happy and comfortable with her surroundings and her coworkers. Her boss was affable, and even malleable at times. Even if she was late in the morning, nothing was said.

She was in a comfort zone that she loved and did not want to change. Later, her boss moved onto another position in the company, and there was a change of personnel.

Her new boss was difficult. He kept Mandy to a timetable, was critical of her work and was scathing to her in front of the other staff. Mandy went into meltdown.

Her comfort zone had completely disappeared and she felt insecure and misplaced. She had made the mistake of assuming that her comfort zone would last forever.

She had limited her life to her comfort zone, and was completely thrown when her situation changed.

Most of us do not actively seek comfort zones. They usually just arise in a situation, and we become lazy and blinkered because we enjoy the feeling of the security it provides us.

Feeling uncomfortable in a situation is never a choice. We would always try to avoid it. Our subconscious mind will try to protect us from situations that we feel uncomfortable in.

www.TheHiddenSecretsofEFT.com

But staying in a comfort zone, will not achieve your deepest desires and help you reach your ultimate goals.

Please tap on the following setup phrases…

"Even though I want to stay in the comfort zone where the familiarity gives me a feeling of security and stability, I can love and accept myself anyway, fully and completely. I now choose to stretch my comfort zone so I can welcome more abundance into my life."

"Even though I resist change because I don't like the learning curve involved in a new situation, I can love and accept myself anyway, fully and completely. I now choose to embrace and welcome change into my life. Change gives me an opportunity for growth."

How to Be Adaptable

Being adaptable is a skill worth mastering. When you can enjoy the possibility and welcome the fact that things will probably not remain the same, you'll be able to embrace life to the fullest.

It is up to you how you choose to view things. A change in lifestyle due to economic changes, a break-up of a marriage and changes in employment can either be devastating or exciting—depending on your outlook.

If you want to change, train yourself to adapt to new situations. Allow other positive feelings in, rather than the limiting beliefs you have become programmed to accept.

Please tap on the following setup phrases…

"Even though I am just not an adaptable kind of person (that's just not my personality), I can love and accept myself anyway, fully and completely. I now choose to be open to being more adaptable in small ways increasing my comfort zone every day."

"Even though I have believed my security came from things staying constant and the same, I can love and accept myself anyway, fully and completely. I now choose to believe that security comes from inside me and not from external circumstances."

"Even though I have always viewed change in the worst possible light, I can love and accept myself anyway, fully and completely. I now choose to change how I think, so I view change as a positive thought bringing new opportunities."

"Even though it feels safe to stay where I am, I can love and accept myself anyway, fully and completely. I now choose to welcome, instead of resist change."

To become the person you want to be, you must act like that person and really believe you are that person. Eventually, that person is who you will become.

Part of morphing into the person you want to be is being open to new ideas, circumstances and opportunities.

We have all been programmed with limiting beliefs about what we think is acceptable for us. Broaden your thinking and become more ambitious in what you choose to undertake.

For example, you could visit places you would never consider going before, eat different foods or take up a new hobby.

If you had unlimited money what would you do? Make a list of all the places and things you would visit and do. You don't have to spend lots of money to access your dreams.

If you have always dreamed of staying in a certain fancy hotel, you can visit the bar there and just have a drink, soaking up the atmosphere.

If you have a dream house in mind, make an appointment to view the house with a real estate agent. They don't have to know you can't afford to buy it yet. It's important you begin to really "feel" yourself living in your dream life.

While you are carrying out your plan, it is likely that certain emotions will rise to the surface. Tap on any emotions such as fear, resentment or discomfort. If you are serious about living your dream life you must take action and clear any discomfort.

Use the following setup phrases as examples for tapping on your own discomfort…

> *"Even though I can't possibly act like the person I want to be because it doesn't feel comfortable, I can love and accept myself anyway, fully and completely. I now choose to accept and move through my discomfort with grace."*
>
> *"Even though I have limited myself, by accepting my life how it is and not believing I am worthy of more, I can love and accept myself anyway, fully and completely. I now choose to*

forgive myself, trusting that any desires I have can be a reality and are not just far-fetched dreams."

"Even though I felt like a fraud when I viewed my dream house that I can't afford yet, I can love and accept myself anyway, fully and completely. I now choose to trust that, part of the process of attaining my dream house is feeling confident and trusting around the idea."

"Even though my family thought I was crazy and didn't understand why I wanted to visit my dream house, I can love and accept myself anyway, fully and completely. I now choose to trust myself and not listen to those who try to drag me down, even if they are my family."

"Even though I didn't belong in the hotel bar and even felt intimidated by the reception staff, I can love and accept myself anyway, fully and completely. I now choose to be proud of myself for stepping out of my comfort zone knowing the more I do this the more confident I will feel."

"Even though I felt worthless test-driving the car, as the car salesman viewed me as a time-waster, I can love and accept myself anyway, fully and completely. I now choose to be proud of myself for stepping out of my comfort zone, knowing the more I do this the more confident I will feel."

"Even though I don't want to ask the price of something because they may get annoyed if I don't actually purchase it, I can love and accept myself anyway, fully and completely. I now choose to accept that it is my decision whether I buy something or not, and I won't be pressured into anything."

www.TheHiddenSecretsofEFT.com

"Even though in the past I've felt I don't deserve and don't belong in the experiences I desire, I can love and accept myself anyway, fully and completely. I now choose to feel more and more comfortable with the situations, people and possessions I desire, knowing these are my divine right."

"Even though I feel resentful that I can't live my dreams right now, I can love and accept myself anyway, fully and completely. I now choose to be patient, knowing that each step I take is bringing me closer towards my goals."

Life is an Adventure

As we have discussed, life can present many opportunities to you. It is important that you have goals you can focus on and are striving towards. It is up to you to decide what you want to experience, enjoy and achieve.

It is also important you don't become blind to opportunities and recognize them for exactly what they are.

For instance, if you perceive your life as being undermined by the amount of money you earn, means that opportunities may come and go. You may not have recognized them because you have felt that those opportunities were not meant for you.

Removing this block will open your mind to the freedom of new thoughts and ideas.

We have already said that the Universe looks after us all. However, before we can assume that we will be on the

Universe's list to receive abundance, we must be open to abundance from various channels and give thanks to all gifts of life.

Accept even the smallest gift with gratitude. Be grateful when someone in the street smiles at you. Or when you receive great customer service in a store. Be thankful there was a cab waiting for you at the stand, when usually there would be none.

In Buddhist thinking, you are advised to "wear the cloak of life loosely." This means you should walk, talk and act freely with confidence and joy. If you are not already living like this, use EFT to loosen your own cloak.

Please tap on the following setup phrases…

> *"Even though there is still a part of me that doesn't believe I can live my dreams, I can love and accept myself anyway, fully and completely. I now choose to be open to my limiting beliefs and dissolve them one by one."*

> *"Even though opportunities are meant for other people and not me, I can love and accept myself anyway, fully and completely. I now choose to forgive myself knowing that I too am as deserving of seizing opportunities as anyone else."*

> *"Even though I don't believe the Universe is on my side, as I've always been dealt a bad hand, I can love and accept myself anyway, fully and completely. I now choose to accept that whatever I believe will become my reality whether my beliefs are negative or positive."*

"Even though I have failed to see the wealth of abundance surrounding me, I can love and accept myself anyway, fully and completely. I now choose to open my eyes and be grateful for all that is bestowed upon me."

"Even though I have been closed to the infinite wealth surrounding me, I can love and accept myself anyway, fully and completely. I now choose to be open to the many diverse channels of abundance—whether they are known or unknown—with complete gratitude."

www.TheHiddenSecretsofEFT.com

Case Study

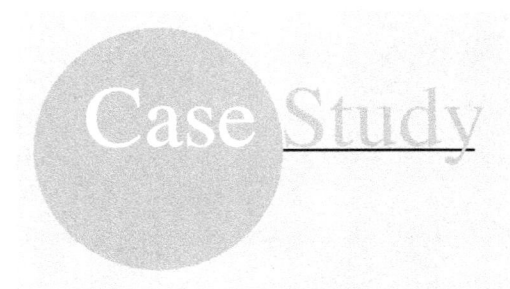

I had one particular client who wanted to work on creating more wealth in her life.

Once we started tapping, we realized there were multiple layers and aspects to the problem.

Initially we started tapping on...

"Even though I'm not sure why I resist making more money, perhaps I can open my mind up to finding the reason, so that I can clear it."

After tapping for just one round on *"not sure why"* and *"opening up my mind"* she had a thought she had never realized before about her husband.

So we then started tapping on...

"Even though I'm afraid that if I make more money than my husband he will resent me, I love and accept myself anyway and now choose to feel calm and comfortable with earning more."

After a few rounds of tapping on *"this fear of him resenting me,"* she realized that there was also a connection with her mother.

Next we tapped on…

"Even though my mother is really negative and tells me I won't be able to earn a full-time income with my business, I love and accept myself anyway and choose to see my unlimited potential."

She was then able to feel like her mother's comments didn't affect her at all.

However, when asked *"what was the upside of earning less money or the downside of earning more,"* she realized some important aspects.

She knew she was more comfortable with earning less money, but felt a lot of pressure with the idea of earning more (as people would then expect more of her).

So we tapped on the following…

"Even though I'm comfortable with earning the income I've always earned, I love and accept myself anyway and now choose to see that I am worthy and deserving of a higher income."

We also tapped on…

"Even though I feel a lot of pressure when I think of earning more money, I love and accept myself anyway; and now choose to feel calm and confident when it comes to earning more money."

www.TheHiddenSecretsofEFT.com

I then asked her to think of another woman that she knew of, that was already earning the desired income my client was after. I asked my client to notice how she felt when she thought of this woman and that amount of income.

My client noticed she felt like she didn't deserve the money, and that it wasn't something that was possible for her.

The tapping continued with…

"Even though I feel like I don't deserve to earn that much, I love and accept myself anyway; and now choose to feel that I do deserve to earn that much."

"Even though it seems like she can earn that much money but not me, I love and accept myself anyway; and choose to feel that if she can do it, so can I."

Finally, when I asked her how she felt about having her business as her only source of income (because she was also working at a part-time job for stability, and wanted to quit), she instantly felt nervous.

So we tapped on the remaining aspects…

"Even though I feel nervous about quitting my job and the financial instability that might result, I choose instead to feel calm and confident and trust that I can do this."

"Even though I feel nervous about having my business as my only source of income, I love and accept myself anyway. I now choose to trust that my business can provide me with more income than I could possibly need."

And finally this remaining aspect...

"Even though I'm afraid of allowing my business to grow because of what others might think of me, I love and accept myself anyway, fully and completely. I choose instead to release this fear."

After this we were not able to find any more aspects to tap on for that particular session.

However, I felt more aspects would crop up, as her life would begin to change.

Please note, tapping on 10 different aspects is a basic minimum for most complex issues.

www.TheHiddenSecretsofEFT.com

Creating Your New Identity

"Nobody can go back and start a new beginning, but anyone can start today and make a new ending."
~ Maria Robinson

www.TheHiddenSecretsofEFT.com

Creating the Identity You Desire

We all know how we would like to be. There are certain personalities or identities that we envy. Yet our beliefs about ourselves limit the possibility of us changing.

Luckily EFT is a great tool that can enable us to become the people we want to be.

We are usually happier to talk about the negative aspects of our lives rather than the positive.

When asked who and how we would like to be, how would we usually answer?

Please tap on any of the following setup phrases that apply to you and use them as examples to create your own...

"Even though I tell myself that I do the best I can, but it's not what I really want, I can love and accept myself anyway, fully and completely. I now choose to be open to expecting and deserving the highest and best in life."

"Even though I should be grateful I even have a job—despite not liking it, I can love and accept myself anyway, fully and completely. I now choose to actively look for a job I know I'll enjoy, because I deserve to be happy in my job."

"Even though I'll never have a lot of money for _____ (I'm just not the type), I can love and accept myself anyway, fully and completely. I now choose to believe I am as deserving as anyone else at being rich."

> *"Even though my family think I'm a "no hoper" (and they're probably right), I can love and accept myself anyway, fully and completely. I now choose to strive for a more positive attitude as my beliefs shape my life."*
>
> *"Even though I'm so unfit and not particularly healthy, I can love and accept myself anyway, fully and completely. I now choose to be open to actively changing my thoughts and lifestyle."*
>
> *"Even though I'm too old and it's too late for me to go after what I really want, I can love and accept myself anyway, fully and completely. I now choose to be open to more adventure, enjoyment and new experiences."*

To begin to change your life you must begin with your thinking. It is lazy and extremely negative to keep telling yourself these limiting phrases.

Most of us want to strive, achieve and be more—whether you want more respect, adventure or fun, or whether you want more money, joy or loving relationships.

This is the purpose of life—to strive for more happiness.

By changing your negative emotions and beliefs, you will free yourself and generate greater abundance and a better life. Please tap on the following setup phrases…

> *"Even though I have been lazy and indulged in negative thinking, I can love and accept myself anyway, fully and completely. I now choose to be more conscious of my thoughts and substitute them for more positive thoughts."*

"Even though I don't believe that if I change my thinking I can change my world, I can love and accept myself anyway, fully and completely. I now choose to realize the truth—that thoughts become words, they become actions, and in turn, I have experiences that create my life."

How Do You Describe Yourself?

If someone were to ask you to describe yourself, what would you say?

Take all the things you automatically say (these will most likely be negative) and then re-phrase them into positive statements.

For example, if you say you are someone who doesn't have a lot of money. Then turn this statement into: *"I am worthy of having more money than I can spend."*

If you automatically say you don't get what you want in life. Then turn this statement into: *"I am capable of achieving all my goals and more."*

If you tell yourself you are unhealthy and unfit. Then turn this statement into: *"I am becoming more physically fit and healthy each day."*

If you describe yourself as someone who always has dramas in their life, then turn this statement into: *"I am at peace with myself and everyone in it."*

These statements are useful for you to change your current thoughts. Say them and believe them while carrying out rounds of tapping on each one. Ensure they're phrased in the present tense.

If these statements don't feel real or true to you, then take note of what emotions arise. Create new setup statements that your brain can accept, and then tap away any negative emotions that arise.

Now is the Time to Act

When you are comfortable that you are in the right position to act, you must do so.

Thinking, saying and affirming is incredibly important to the changes we wish to make in our lives.

But without action, they are meaningless. They become hazy dreams that never eventuate, because you didn't act upon them.

What is preventing you from taking action? Please be honest with yourself. It may be one big fear, or a combination of all of the above.

Are you scared of hard work? Do you think the world owes you, and your goals should magically manifest from the sky into your lap without you lifting a finger?

Do you keep putting it off and off, thinking you will start on your goal another day? Have you procrastinated for as long as you can remember?

Are you frightened of the consequences of your actions,

and the inevitable change that will come with achieving that goal?

Are you frightened you may fail and not achieve your goal? Failure, is the ultimate humiliation for some people–it scares them so much, they don't even bother to try.

Are you scared of the success that will manifest in your life as a result of realizing that goal?

Are you scared of the new responsibility that reaching your goal will involve?

Are you scared of losing friends or family? Do you think achieving your goal will alienate you from your loved ones?

Let's have a look in detail at all of the above fears.

Fear of Hard Work

Every single person who has ever achieved their goals, has worked hard for them. They didn't sit around complaining about their lives, they did something about it.

Do you feel someone else should achieve your goals for you? Do you expect financial hand-outs from your parents when you are an adult? Do you expect your husband to be responsible for providing you with your dream home?

The world doesn't owe you anything. You owe it to yourself to create your life how you want it to be.

Please tap on the following setup statements…

"Even though I don't believe I have to work hard for the things I want in life, I can love and accept myself anyway, fully and completely. I now choose to accept that I am responsible for my life."

"Even though I expect others and the world to provide me with my goals on a silver platter, I can love and accept myself anyway, fully and completely. I now choose to realize I've been provided with the opportunity to realize my goals myself."

"Even though I am unwilling to work hard for my dreams, I can love and accept myself anyway, fully and completely. I now choose to be open to the idea that my dreams will never materialize without effort from me."

Procrastination

Avoiding action through procrastination has its roots in fear. Many people who procrastinate are in fact perfectionists.

Are you one of these people who cannot begin anything until everything is in order? Do you fear that if you can't control every situation, something may happen that you may not be able to deal with?

Unfortunately, the need for a perfect situation paralyzes you into doing nothing. Plus, to meet your high standards, you need everything "ready" and sorted, before you get started on your goal. So then your goal never actually gets started.

Please tap on the following setup statements…

"Even though I can't possibly start on my goal because I don't know all the answers, I can love and accept myself anyway, fully and completely. I now choose to trust that the things I need to know will be made clear to me, as I work towards my goal."

"Even though I've wasted so much time worrying about my goals but not doing anything about it, I can love and accept myself anyway, fully and completely. I now choose to forgive myself, and resolve to quell all feelings of future procrastination."

"Even though I'm just waiting for _____ to happen, before I start on my goal, I can love and accept myself anyway, fully and completely. I now choose to start on my goal, and be open to the fact that things don't have to happen in the exact order I think they should."

"Even though I'd rather not do it at all than make a mistake, I can love and accept myself anyway, fully and completely. I now choose to accept that it is only human and natural to make mistakes, and there is nothing wrong with making lots of mistakes."

"Even though it's been so hard for me to take action towards my goals, I can love and accept myself anyway, fully and completely. I now choose to take action when most appropriate—without unnecessary delay; easily and consistently."

Please list all the reasons why you find it difficult to get started. Create setup statements out of your limiting beliefs and then clear these feelings with EFT.

Fear of Change

Continuing with the same behaviors, will not change the results you are achieving. Taking the same path will get you to the same place over and over.

This quote, attributed to Albert Einstein: "The definition of insanity is continuing to do the same thing over and over, and then expecting different results," reinforces that you won't get anywhere taking the same path, and suggests you may end up insane in the process!

The only way you can reach the results you want is by doing everything differently. Thinking differently, speaking differently and acting differently.

Unless you are prepared to change things, your ultimate result will be the same.

Perhaps you want to lose weight, yet you're not prepared to eat healthier foods or exercise more. You want to stop smoking and yet you continue to buy cigarettes. You dislike your job and yet you don't make the time or effort to find something different. Much of this is due to fear of change.

If you recognize any of the above stopping you from moving forward in your own life, then please tap on the following setup statements…

"Even though acting in a different way feels scary to me, I can love and accept myself anyway, fully and completely. I now choose to stretch my comfort zone and embrace the unknown."

"Even though I'd rather stay where I am, because I am so worried about what may or may not happen if I change what I already know, I can love and accept myself anyway, fully and completely. I now choose to risk living the life I've always desired, by making the effort to go after what I really want."

"Even though I've been approved for a mortgage, but part of me doubts I'll be able to meet the monthly repayments, I can love and accept myself anyway, fully and completely. I now choose to trust that the Universe will support me in realizing my dreams, if I take the first step towards them."

"Even though I fear not knowing how I will cope once I begin something, I can love and accept myself anyway, fully and completely. I now choose to trust that whatever solutions I need, will make themselves known to me at the time I need them."

"Even though there is still part of me that fears change in some way, I can love and accept myself anyway, fully and completely. I now choose to take new actions and see where I am led."

Fear of Failure

The experience of failure can be difficult to put behind you, and it can color everything you subsequently undertake.

Fear of failure can be one of the biggest stumbling blocks to your own success. Perhaps you fear failing, so you don't even bother starting. Or you may fear failing, and you find a reason to sabotage your efforts just when you are nearing completion of your goal.

Perhaps a past incident where you have failed comes back to haunt you in your new goals. It's important you don't let past events rule how you act today.

Feelings of childhood failure can be a very emotional experience that can remain with you, and will easily override any adult logic.

Please tap on the following setup statements…

> *"Even though I don't want to put myself in any situation where I could fail because I've failed in the past and it was so painful, I can love and accept myself anyway, fully and completely. I now choose to accept that failing is part of the process to achieving my goals."*

> *"Even though I am scared to try new things and like to stay safely within experiences that I know, I can love and accept myself anyway, fully and completely. I now choose to try new things and break through my safety barriers."*

"Even though I have feared failing for so long I can love and accept myself anyway, fully and completely. I now choose to feel confident and view each outcome as part of the learning curve, be it successful or not."

Return to your childhood and relive any memories where you experienced negative emotions due to failing.

Perhaps your Dad put you down no matter what you did (and no matter how hard you tried). Perhaps a teacher once told you that only losers make mistakes (and you felt you must be a loser as you made a small mistake).

Perhaps a friend of your parents told you that at your age you should be able to swim, and didn't believe you when you told them you couldn't.

Perhaps your Mom repeated time and time again to get something right the first time or not to bother with it at all (that made you afraid to even attempt something, for fear of not doing it perfectly).

Whatever experiences you have of failure, it's important you rectify them so you can move forward freely with your life.

Do not feel embarrassed or feel your experiences are trivial. Your emotions related to those experiences are very real, and must be treated with respect and not downplayed.

Fear of Success

It seems like a contradiction that you may be scared or frightened of succeeding at something you want in your life.

Being successful may be an emotion you are not used to experiencing. It can change lives, forcing you into situations where you need to make more decisions and apply new pressures (especially if it is business success).

The achievement of one goal can affect your whole life.

Nelson Mandela addressed this issue in his Inaugural Speech in 1994 when he recited:

Our Greatest Fear

Our greatest fear is not that we are inadequate,
but that we are powerful beyond measure.

It is our light, not our darkness, that frightens us.

We ask ourselves, who am I to be brilliant,
gorgeous, handsome, talented and fabulous?

Actually, who are you not to be?

You are a child of God.

Your playing small does not serve the world.

There is nothing enlightened about shrinking,
so that other people won't feel insecure around you.

We were born to make manifest the glory of God within us.

It is not just in some; it is in everyone.

As we let our own light shine, we consciously give other people permission to do the same.

As we are liberated from our fear, our presence automatically liberates others."

Marianne Williamson from her book *A Return to Love*.

Please use the following setup statements to tap on the following potential trappings of success...

"Even though I would rather be comfortable than succeed, I can love and accept myself anyway, fully and completely. I now choose to be open to succeeding and accept, that feeling uncomfortable is only a temporary feeling until I adjust."

"Even though being successful is seen as a negative, greedy trait by my family, I can love and accept myself anyway, fully and completely. I now choose to allow my family to think what they choose. I choose to respect, instead of resent those who have achieved success."

"Even though I've always believed "blowing your own trumpet" was bad, and I associate being successful is like blowing your own trumpet, I can love and accept myself anyway, fully and completely. I now choose to realize it is silly to downplay the goals I have worked hard to achieve."

"Even though I don't want to be successful—as I view success as having more pitfalls than positives, I can love and accept myself anyway, fully and completely. I now choose to change my beliefs about what success means to me."

www.TheHiddenSecretsofEFT.com

"Even though I don't want to be successful because successful people are always bust, and I'll have no time for my family, I can love and accept myself anyway, fully and completely. I now choose to believe the opposite—that being successful will allow me the freedom to spend even more time with my family."

"Even though I have feared the consequences of my potential success, I can love and accept myself anyway, fully and completely. I now choose to let go of this fear and allow myself to experience the highest levels of success in all areas of my life."

Write down your thoughts, attitudes and experiences surrounding success.

Look at people you know who have already achieved a level of success that you would like to be at, and ask yourself what you think of these people?

Look at celebrity success stories and ask yourself what you think of these personalities?

If any of your thoughts are negative you need to clear them with EFT.

After you have done this, make a list of the goals and dreams that you have listed, but not yet achieved in your life. What excuses come up as to why you have not achieved them?

Please create setup statements out of your excuses and use EFT to tap on them until all negativity is resolved.

Fear of Responsibility

Sometimes it's easier to point the finger and blame the world for the things that haven't happened, than to actively take responsibility for your own life.

Do you blame the world's economic crisis for the fact you lost your job? Do you blame your parents for being overweight and out of shape because you inherited their genes?

It is time to stop accusing the world for your own shortcomings and take matters into your own hands.

It is true that we were not all born equal. The amount of opportunities available to us depends on the circumstances and willingness of our family and their friends.

But it is a fact that even those born into the most derelict and deprived circumstances can achieve success in their lives.

Pick up any autobiography of any famous person and see for yourself. It is likely they overcame huge obstacles before realizing their success.

Please use the following setup phrases as examples of any fears surrounding responsibility you may have...

> "Even though I have become so used to blaming everyone but myself for all the disappointments, failures and shortcomings in my life, I can love and accept myself anyway, fully and completely. I now choose to accept with gratitude the power I have in creating the life exactly how I would like it."

"Even though I feel burdened by the responsibility for making my life how I want it, I can love and accept myself anyway, fully and completely. I now choose to recognize and be grateful for the freedom and multiple choices I have in how I live my life."

"Even though I don't want to be too good at my job because I don't want to deal with the pressure of accepting a higher position with increased responsibility, I can love and accept myself anyway, fully and completely. I now choose to accept I am worthy and capable of new responsibilities, and look forward to a higher position."

"Even though I have not owned my thoughts, words and actions in the past I can love and accept myself anyway, fully and completely. I now choose to forgive myself and everyone I've pointed a finger at."

"Even though I believe rich people are often stressed out and I don't want to be stressed out if I become rich, I can love and accept myself anyway, fully and completely. I now choose to accept that if I look after my money, I will not become stressed because of it."

"Even though I won't know what to do with large amounts of money and I feel afraid, I can love and accept myself anyway, fully and completely. I now choose to accept that as long as I feel afraid of money it will never come to me."

"Even though I'm scared of making a lot of money, because that requires increased responsibility, I can love and accept myself anyway, fully and completely. I now choose to be *open to learning how to manage and nurture large sums of money and become comfortable with it."*

Fear of Losing Friends and Family

If you have ever felt hatred, jealousy or resentment towards other people and their wealth and success—it is likely you believe others will feel those same things about you when you become wealthy.

Some of your deep-rooted needs will include feeling liked and accepted by other people. If you know that having a lot of money will alienate those close to you, then you will subconsciously find ways not to achieve wealth (even though you may still desire it).

If you believe having great abundance or success in your life will make you feel uncomfortable, left out and different; then you may end up sabotaging your own efforts of reaching your goals. The reason being, part of you doesn't want to deal with the consequences.

It's useful to think about who would feel threatened when you achieved your chosen goals. Would your partner feel threatened if you made more money than them?

Will your circle of friends feel jealous of you when you live in your dream house with an enviable lifestyle?

List all your fears regarding past and likely future rejections and abandonment from those you love, and turn them into setup phrases to tap on. Please use the following setup phrases as examples of fears related to losing family and friends if you become successful…

> "Even though my friends will reject me and I'll be socially outcast if I make significantly more money than them, I can love and accept myself anyway, fully and completely. I now choose to realize that true friends will stick by me and celebrate in my success."

> "Even though if I earn more money than my Dad he won't love me anymore as he will feel inferior, I can love and accept myself anyway, fully and completely. I now choose to accept that I cannot sacrifice living my life to please my Dad, and that my dreams are worth more than his blessing."

> "Even though I'm afraid to buy the new car I like as my neighbors will think I'm showing off, I can love and accept myself anyway, fully and completely. I now choose to believe that I can't please everyone so I may as well please myself."

> "Even though society hates rich and successful people (and I don't want to be disliked by society), I can love and accept myself anyway, fully and completely. I now choose to accept there are many generous, kind and loving people in this world who are rich and successful."

> "Even though I have been abandoned in the past (which has led me to avoid situations where this rejection may happen again), I can love and accept myself anyway, fully and completely. I now choose to forgive myself and those involved. I now trust that those around me will now support me and any changes in my life."

Fear of Commitment

There is boldness in committing strongly to your dreams. Commitment means that you will do everything in your power until you reach your dreams—no matter what!

It doesn't mean you give up when you come to your first obstacle. It doesn't mean that you complain what you are doing is too hard. And it doesn't mean you are so narrow-minded you refuse to be flexible about changing the nature of your goal.

If you are serious about changing your life for the better, commit your goals to paper. Jot down when you would like to realize your goals by. Take each big goal and break it down into manageable steps.

Get started on your goals—the first journey begins with a single step. Don't wait for tomorrow, start today!

Please tap on the following setup phrases if you are feeling any resistance towards committing to your goals...

"Even though I am scared to commit to my goals because I may not achieve them and then I'll look foolish, I can love and accept myself anyway, fully and completely. I now choose to decide whether I tell anyone else about my goals or not, recognizing there is power in being silent in some cases."

"Even though I've never committed to anything before in my life, I can love and accept myself anyway, fully and completely. I now choose to accept there is a first time for everything and that the time to commit to my goals is today."

www.TheHiddenSecretsofEFT.com

"Even though there is something inside me that is preventing me from committing to my goals, I can love and accept myself anyway, fully and completely. I now choose to be open to what this block may be so I can dissolve it with EFT."

"Even though I have a tendency to give up easily I can love and accept myself anyway, fully and completely. I now choose to recognize the stage I'd normally give up at and persevere anyway."

"Even though my goal is way too hard for me to finish, I can love and accept myself anyway, fully and completely. I now choose to accept that everyone who achieved anything worthwhile, worked hard for it. I am now willing to show the same courage and persistence."

Have Faith and Believe in Yourself

There is no point striving towards a goal if you don't believe in your heart that you can do it.

The power is in your hands and you can choose to go for your goals 100% or not. No one can give you faith. Others can encourage and cheer you on, but only you can believe in yourself.

There are some people who naturally seem to have more confidence and trust in themselves than others do.

Perhaps you may have had numerous bad experiences in your past that have clouded how you view the world. If you are one of these people please use EFT to resolve any emotional resistance.

Do not settle for your life being mediocre. You were born to dream, aspire and reach for more. Now is the time to live, accept and enjoy success in all areas of your life.

Please tap on the following setup phrases removing any fears related to the confidence you have in your own abilities...

"Even though I have zero confidence in myself or my abilities to create the life I desire, I can love and accept myself anyway, fully and completely. I now choose to forgive myself and have complete faith I can succeed in reaching my goals."

"Even though I have been conditioned to accept my life being satisfactory and as the best I can do, I can love and accept myself anyway, fully and completely. I now choose to turn my back on mediocrity and reach for full satisfaction in every area of my life."

"Even though I have believed it was wrong to go after my dreams because I'm not the "success type", I can love and accept myself anyway, fully and completely. I now choose to forgive myself and anyone else involved. I now accept everyone is worthy of aiming for their dreams, including me."

"Even though I have not trusted other people because in the past I have been badly let down, I can love and accept myself anyway, fully and completely. I now choose to be open to trusting people again, knowing I cannot reach my goals without enlisting the support of others."

"Even though I have never had any faith in the Universe to provide me with opportunities I need to reach my goals, I can love and accept myself anyway, fully and completely. I now choose to forgive myself and trust that all the opportunities I could hope for will be made available to me when I need them."

Patience: Allowing Time to Change

Now that you have confidence in yourself to achieve your goals, it is time to exercise some patience.

Impatience demonstrates a lack of trust. Some goals take longer than others to manifest. The trick is to keep persisting, knowing that you will realize your goals if you keep going.

Often the "darkest" period is just before your goals materialize. This is unfortunately the time most people give up. We need to recognize this period and persevere more than ever.

The time when you feel like giving up most is definitely not the time to stop! Keep going as your goals are most likely just around the corner…

In fact, many successful people talk of a particularly difficult time when they felt like giving up—but they didn't. And luckily for them they didn't because shortly after they achieved their goals.

Being methodical and consistent will see you through to your goals.

You need to know that the changes you desire in your life will not be instant. Right now you are still living your life through your existing beliefs—many of which will be slowing you down.

Persistence is required to change the thoughts, habits and beliefs that have accompanied you during your lifetime.

Please tap on the following setup phrases...

"Even though I want everything in my whole life to change immediately, I can love and accept myself anyway, fully and completely. I now choose to be patient and learn the lessons I need to learn along the path to my goals."

"Even though there is part of me that doesn't trust my goals will ever eventuate as it is taking too long, I can love and accept myself anyway, fully and completely. I now choose to exercise patience and keep going no matter how long it takes, knowing I will get there in the end."

"Even though I've never seen anything through to the end because I'm so impatient, I can love and accept myself anyway, fully and completely. I now choose to keep persisting until I reach my goals."

"Even though I have kept on track with my goals but I'm now experiencing an extremely rough patch, I can love and accept myself anyway, fully and completely. I now choose to keep going knowing that very soon I shall reach my goals."

www.TheHiddenSecretsofEFT.com

"Even though I feel like giving up on my goals right now, I can love and accept myself anyway, fully and completely. I now choose to move slowly and deliberately through my resistance and realize my goals."

Creating New Ways of Thinking

If after persevering you are not currently achieving your goals, then perhaps it's time to look at a new way of getting there.

You would have heard the phrase, "think outside the box"? Well, finding different ways of changing what you're doing will help you break away from your normal and habitual patterns of thinking so new ideas can come to you.

Please tap on the following setup phrases…

"Even though I can't see a solution or path to achieve my goals, I can love and accept myself anyway, fully and completely. I now choose to change how I think so my mind can provide me with new solutions."

"Even though I am stuck and don't know how to proceed, I can love and accept myself anyway, fully and completely. I now choose to experience effective and creative solutions for every situation I encounter."

"Even though I feel like a failure for not being able to achieve my goals, I can love and accept myself anyway, fully and completely. I now choose to forgive myself and accept a flow of excellent possibilities, that suit my needs perfectly."

www.TheHiddenSecretsofEFT.com

Case Study

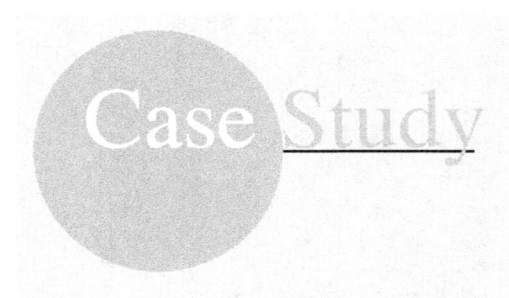

A good example of helping someone to create a new identity with EFT, was one woman in particular that I worked with that always saw herself as a victim and had a "victim identity".

EFT worked beautifully to clear all the aspects connected to her victim identity, and with continual work, she was able to take on the identity of someone who was empowered to change and create her own life.

The session started with her feeling frustrated with her marriage and financial situation and helpless to change it.

We started tapping on...

> *"Even though I'm really frustrated with my husband and his lack of financial support, I choose now to let this feeling go and open up my mind to see the situation differently."*

Then we tapped on...

> *"Even though I'm frustrated because it feels like there is nothing I can do to change my situation, I choose now to let this frustration go and open up my mind to find a solution to the problem."*

And then we tapped on…

"Even though I feel helpless to change our financial situation, I love and accept myself anyway; and choose to let that helpless feeling go and feel empowered instead."

In alignment with my client's victim mentality, she explained that she was already working long hours at two different jobs, and feeling exhausted and burnt out.

She explained that their financial problems were her husband's fault, as he refused to get out of his sales job that only provided very inconsistent income.

We then tapped on…

"Even though I want to blame my husband for all of our financial problems, maybe I can choose to see the situation differently and allow myself to find a way to work with my husband instead."

Then we tapped on…

"Even though I feel burnt out and exhausted, I love and accept myself anyway and choose now to give myself permission to relax no matter what."

And then we tapped on…

"Even though I've been under this constant financial stress and pressure, I choose now to let go of this stress and feel calm and relaxed instead."

My client also explained that she had many other responsibilities in her life, and had no time to take care of her own needs, that made her feel helpless in changing.

So we tapped on...

"Even though I'm angry that there seems to be no time for me and take care of my own needs, I love and accept myself anyway, and I choose now to be open to changing that pattern."

And then we tapped on...

"Even though I'm exhausted with all these responsibilities in my life, and feel helpless in changing them; I choose now to restore my energy and feel empowered to change my life instead."

At this point, I asked my client *"what did this helpless feeling remind her of"* and *"what was her earliest memory of this same feeling."*

She started to cry, as she realized that she had felt this way almost her whole life, ever since she was a child.

She explained that after her parents separated, she was responsible for many things in the home, at school and felt helpless to change any of it.

This allowed us to begin tapping on the root issue...

"Even though there were too many responsibilities placed upon me by my parents when I was a child, I love and accept myself anyway and give myself permission to see

the situation differently now."

Then we tapped on...

"Even though I feel like I've been helpless to change my circumstances since I was a child, I love and accept myself anyway, fully and completely. Instead, I choose now to feel empowered to change my life."

"Even though I felt like a victim surrounding my circumstances as a child, I love and accept myself anyway and choose now to see the situation differently."

And then we tapped on...

"Even though being a victim has become part of my identity and it's really scary to let that go, I choose now to let that fear go and allow myself to take on a new identity as an empowered woman."

My client then realized that there were some more feelings about changing her identity as being a helpless victim in her circumstances, to an empowered woman who created her own life.

So we finished by tapping on...

"Even though I feel overwhelmed by the responsibility for making my life how I want it, I love and accept myself anyway, and choose instead to feel blessed with the opportunity to create my life the way I want it."

And then we finally tapped on:

"Even though I don't think it's possible for me to really let

go of my victim identity, I love, accept and forgive myself anyway. I choose now to open up my mind to see that it is possible for me in so many ways."

Our session ended with my client understanding that it was time to let go of her victim identity and that it would feel so much better to take charge of her life direction.

Changing your identity with EFT, definitely requires finding the root issues, and the time in your life when the identity was created. Once this is done, infinite possibilities lie ahead to create a whole new identity for yourself.

www.TheHiddenSecretsofEFT.com

Final Thoughts

"Freedom is not worth having if it does not include the freedom to make mistakes."
~ Mahatma Gandhi

www.TheHiddenSecretsofEFT.com

Final Thoughts...

EFT is the most powerful tool I've come across to change your life. It's empowering because it is a relatively easy skill to learn, and then put into practice.

The measure of how well you've grasped EFT, will be evident in the results you see in your life every day.

A client of mine summed it up nicely when she told me she thought it was necessary to have strong emotions attached to memories. She was relieved when she discovered that she could feel neutral about certain incidents in her past that previously upset her.

The beauty of EFT is in its power to penetrate to the root cause of virtually any issue you have. True emotional freedom is the experience of releasing any negative emotions associated with a particular belief.

There is no right or wrong time-frame to use EFT. Many people experience instant results—some people may take longer.

It's worth sharing that those who do experience "instant results" are honest about what they are feeling. Many people are afraid to be completely honest—even with themselves. If this is your situation, I encourage you to release this block first before using EFT on other things you wish to change.

It is my desire that you personally adopt and adapt EFT for your own personal use, and that you call upon EFT throughout your life whenever you need it.

www.TheHiddenSecretsofEFT.com

Remember, if you get really stuck, there are many EFT Therapists that you can call on to assist you on your healing journey—just look up a practitioner in your local area.

I trust you will have as many brilliant and transformative results as I have experienced with EFT.

Many blessings on your journey to freedom.

~ Carol Prentice

www.TheHiddenSecretsofEFT.com

www.TheHiddenSecretsofEFT.com

How to Access Your 3 FREE EFT Training Videos

I encourage you to watch EFT in action as well as read about it. Most of us are visual people who absorb a lot, simply by watching.

This is why I've created an **Online EFT Training Series** compromising of 23 videos (19 hours, 57 minutes) you can watch online.

To see if the **Online EFT Training Series** is right for you, I'm giving readers FREE access to watch 3 videos of individuals using EFT to dissolve their issues.

You will benefit from watching if you can relate to any of the following...

- Feel ashamed and embarrassed about yourself because of how you look (and no matter how hard you try, you simply can't accept your body).

- Seek approval from others to validate yourself (because you care more about what others think than you do your own opinion).

- Feel scared to love someone and emotionally distance yourself from the opposite sex (to avoid the potential pain of being rejected).

To access these 3 FREE videos visit:
www.eft4u.net/freeeftvideos